T0226545

Emerging Pathogens

Editors

NAHED ISMAIL
JAMES W. SNYDER
A. WILLIAM PASCULLE

CLINICS IN LABORATORY MEDICINE

www.labmed.theclinics.com

June 2017 • Volume 37 • Number 2

ELSEVIER

1600 John F. Kennedy Boulevard • Suite 1800 • Philadelphia, Pennsylvania, 19103-2899

http://www.theclinics.com

CLINICS IN LABORATORY MEDICINE Volume 37, Number 2
June 2017 ISSN 0272-2712, ISBN-13: 978-0-323-53015-6

Editor: Stacy Eastman
Developmental Editor: Colleen Dietzler

© 2017 Elsevier Inc. All rights reserved.

Reprints. For copies of 100 or more, of articles in this publication, please contact the Commercial Reprints Department, Elsevier Inc., 360 Park Avenue South, New York, New York 10010-1710. Tel. 212-633-3874, Fax: 212-633-3820, E-mail: reprints@elsevier.com.

Clinics in Laboratory Medicine (ISSN 0272-2712) is published quarterly by Elsevier Inc., 360 Park Avenue South, New York, NY 10010-1710. Months of issue are March, June, September, and December. Business and Editorial offices: 1600 John F. Kennedy Blvd., Suite 1800, Philadelphia, PA 19103-2899. Periodicals postage paid at NewYork, NY and additional mailing offices. Subscription prices are $258.00 per year (US individuals), $488.00 per year (US institutions), $100.00 per year (US students), $314.00 per year (Canadian individuals), $593.00 per year (Canadian institutions), $185.00 per year (Canadian students), $402.00 per year (international individuals), $593.00 per year (international institutions), $185.00 (international students). Foreign air speed delivery is included in all Clinics subscription prices. All prices are subject to change without notice. POSTMASTER: Send address changes to *Clinics in Laboratory Medicine*, Elsevier Health Sciences Division, Subscription Customer Service, 3251 Riverport Lane, Maryland Heights, MO 63043. **Customer Service: 1-800-654-2452 (US). From outside of the US and Canada, call 1-314-447-8871. Fax: 1-314-447-8029. E-mail: journalscustomerservice-usa@elsevier.com (for print support) or journalsonlinesupport-usa@elsevier.com (for online support).**

Clinics in Laboratory Medicine is covered in *EMBASE/Exerpta Medica, MEDLINE/PubMed (Index Medicus), Cinahl, Current Contents/Clinical Medicine, BIOSIS* and *ISI/BIOMED.*

Contributors

EDITORS

NAHED ISMAIL, MD, PhD, D(ABMM), D(ABMLI)
Associate Professor of Pathology and Immunology, Clinical Microbiology Division, University of Pittsburgh, Pittsburgh, Pennsylvania

JAMES W. SNYDER, PhD, D(ABMM), F(AAM)
Director, Microbiology, Department Pathology and Laboratory Medicine, University of Louisville Hospital, Louisville, Kentucky

A. WILLIAM PASCULLE, ScD
Associate Professor of Pathology, Infectious Diseases and Microbiology, Director of Microbiology, University of Pittsburgh Medical Center, Pittsburgh, Pennsylvania

AUTHORS

LUCAS S. BLANTON, MD
Assistant Professor, Infectious Diseases, Department of Internal Medicine, The University of Texas Medical Branch at Galveston, Galveston, Texas

BETHANY G. BOLLING, PhD
Arbovirus Laboratory, Texas Department of State Health Services, Austin, Texas

COLIN S. BROWN, FRCPath
King's Sierra Leone Partnership, King's Centre for Global Health, King's Health Partners, King's College London, National Infection Service, Public Health England, London, United Kingdom

SCOTT R. CURRY, MD
Assistant Professor of Medicine, Division of Infectious Diseases, Medical University of South Carolina, Charleston, South Carolina

YOHEI DOI, MD, PhD
Division of Infectious Diseases, University of Pittsburgh School of Medicine, Pittsburgh, Pennsylvania

RONG FANG, MD, PhD
Assistant Professor, Department of Pathology, The University of Texas Medical Branch at Galveston, Galveston, Texas

AMY HARTMAN, PhD
Assistant Professor, Center for Vaccine Research, Infectious Diseases and Microbiology, University of Pittsburgh Graduate School of Public Health, University of Pittsburgh, Pittsburgh, Pennsylvania

ALINA IOVLEVA, MD
Division of Infectious Diseases, University of Pittsburgh School of Medicine, Pittsburgh, Pennsylvania

NAHED ISMAIL, MD, PhD, D(ABMM), D(ABMLI)
Associate Professor of Pathology and Immunology, Clinical Microbiology Division, University of Pittsburgh, Pittsburgh, Pennsylvania

DONALD JUNGKIND, PhD
Professor and Chair Emeritus, St. George's University School of Medicine, Grenada, West Indies

ANGELLE DESIREE LABEAUD, MD, MS
Associate Professor, Department of Pediatrics, Stanford University School of Medicine, Stanford, California

MICHAEL LOEFFELHOLZ, PhD, D(ABMM)
Director, Clinical Microbiology Laboratory, Professor, Department of Pathology, University of Texas Medical Branch, Galveston, Texas

JERE W. McBRIDE, PhD
Department of Pathology, Center for Biodefense and Emerging Infectious Diseases, Sealy Center for Vaccine Development, University of Texas Medical Branch, Galveston, Texas

STEPHEN MEPHAM, FRCPath
Department of Infection, Royal Free London NHS Foundation Trust, London, United Kingdom

RYAN F. RELICH, PhD, D(ABMM), MLS(ASCP)SM
Assistant Professor, Clinical Pathology and Laboratory Medicine, Medical Director, Clinical Virology and Serology Laboratories, Associate Medical Director, Divisions of Clinical Microbiology and Molecular Pathology, Department of Pathology and Laboratory Medicine, Indiana University School of Medicine, Indiana University Health, Indianapolis, Indiana

VANDANA SAXENA, MSc, PhD
Department of Immunology and Serology, National AIDS Research Institute, Pune, Maharashtra

ROBERT J. SHORTEN, PhD
Public Health Laboratory Manchester, Manchester Royal Infirmary, Manchester, United Kingdom; Department of Infection, Centre for Clinical Microbiology, University College London, London, United Kingdom

DAVID M. VU, MD
Instructor, Department of Pediatrics, Stanford University School of Medicine, Stanford, California

DAVID H. WALKER, MD
The Carmage and Martha Walls Distinguished University Chair in Tropical Diseases, Professor, Department of Pathology, Executive Director, Center for Biodefense and Emerging Infectious Diseases, The University of Texas Medical Branch, Galveston, Texas

TIAN WANG, PhD
Professor, Departments of Microbiology & Immunology, and Pathology, University of Texas Medical Branch, Galveston, Texas

Contents

West Nile virus (WNV) is the most widely distributed flavivirus and causes multiple viral encephalitis outbreaks in humans in different regions worldwide. Nearly half of the WNV convalescent patients are reported to have persistent neurologic sequelae or chronic kidney disease. Neither treatment nor vaccines are available for human use. Current efforts on drug development have mostly been focused on the inhibitors of virus replication. In this review, we discuss recent findings from studies in field and animal models of WNV infection and provide new insights onto WNV transmission, host immunity, viral pathogenesis, diagnosis, and vaccine development.

The ongoing epidemic of Zika fever in the Western Hemisphere has drawn considerable attention from the medical and scientific communities as well as the general public, largely because of its association with birth defects and postinfectious sequelae. Since its appearance in Brazil in 2015, Zika virus has spread to more than 45 countries in the Western Hemisphere and has caused countless infections. To date, no treatment or vaccine exists, but a considerable multinational effort to halt Zika virus transmission is underway. This article reviews the basic biology, epidemiology, pathophysiology, diagnosis, and treatment of Zika virus and Zika fever.

The 2014 to 2016 Ebola virus disease (EVD), through the sheer size of the outbreak and combined experience within both resource-rich and resource-poor settings, allowed for more information to be gained about the clinical and pathologic features of EVD. This review highlights the range of aspects of EVD that the authors find are relevant to laboratory medicine, including the need for robust prediagnostic and laboratory processing algorithms to inform sampling of suspect patients, the vast majority of whom, in resource-rich settings, will have another diagnosis.

the last five years, several new treatment strategies that capitalize on the increasing understanding of the altered microbiome and host defenses in patients with CDI have completed clinical trials, including fecal microbiota transplantation. This article highlights the changing epidemiology, laboratory diagnostics, pathogenesis, and treatment of CDI.

For chikungunya virus (CHIKV), the long-term sequelae from infection are yet ill-defined. The prolonged debilitating arthralgia associated with CHIKV infection has tremendous potential for impacting the global economy and should be considered when evaluating the human burden of disease and the allocation of resources. There is much still unknown about CHIKV and the illnesses that it causes. Developing a better understanding of the pathogenesis of CHIKV infection is a priority and forms the basis for developing effective strategies at infection prevention and disease control.

With advances in molecular genetics, more pathogenic rickettsial species have been identified. Pathogenic rickettsiae are transmitted by vectors, such as arthropods, into the patient's skin and then spread into the microvascular endothelial cells. Clinical manifestations are characterized by fever with headache and myalgias, followed by rash 3 to 5 days later. The undifferentiated nature of clinical symptoms, knowledge of the epidemiology, and the patient's history of travel and exposure to arthropod vectors are critical to the empiric administration of antimicrobial therapy. Doxycycline is currently the most effective antibiotic for treatment of all spotted fever group and typhus group rickettsioses.

CLINICS IN LABORATORY MEDICINE

THE CLINICS ARE NOW AVAILABLE ONLINE!
Access your subscription at:
www.theclinics.com

Preface

 CrossMark

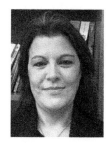 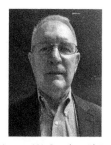 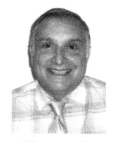

Nahed Ismail, MD, PhD,
D(ABMM), D(ABMLI)

James W. Snyder, PhD,
D(ABMM), F(AAM)

A. William Pasculle, ScD

Editors

Fascination with the incredible diversity and adaptability of microorganisms is what brought many of us to the science of microbiology. These concepts are aptly illuminated in the articles contained herein. Each article, written by those we consider experts in their given fields, gives an overview of the epidemiology and pathogenesis of some of the most important bacterial and viral pathogens of our current times. Some of them, such as Ebola and Zika, are more familiar due to extensive news coverage, while others are less so but equally important. We hope that you, the readers, will find these articles informative and useful.

We understand and appreciate the negative impact that these conditions may have on human health and quality of people's lives. These articles highlight the current scientific information that define each disease, and the serious clinical, diagnostic, preventive, and treatment challenges that need to be addressed through scientific advancement. Although the goal of these articles was not to provide or produce recommendations, we hope that this body of work results in further discussion of research gaps, priorities, and opportunities.

A work such as this is not possible without the collaboration of many individuals. Besides our authors, we are indebted to Lauren Boyle and Colleen Dietzler, the Acquisitions and Developmental Editors at Elsevier.

Nahed Ismail, MD, PhD, D(ABMM), D(ABMLI)
Clinical Microbiology Division
University of Pittsburgh
UPMC Clinical Laboratory Building
3477 Euler Way
Pittsburgh, PA 15213, USA

James W. Snyder, PhD, D(ABMM), F(AAM)
Department of Pathology and Laboratory Medicine
University of Louisville Hospital
530 South Jackson Street
Louisville, KY 40202, USA

Clin Lab Med 37 (2017) ix–x
http://dx.doi.org/10.1016/j.cll.2017.03.001
0272-2712/17/© 2017 Published by Elsevier Inc.

labmed.theclinics.com

A. William Pasculle, ScD
University of Pittsburgh Medical Center
Pittsburgh, PA 15237, USA

E-mail addresses:
ismailn@upmc.edu (N. Ismail)
james.snyder@louisville.edu (J.W. Snyder)
pasculleaw@upmc.edu (A.W. Pasculle)

West Nile Virus

Vandana Saxena, MSc, PhD[a], Bethany G. Bolling, PhD[b],
Tian Wang, PhD[c,d,]*

KEYWORDS

- West Nile virus • Flavivirus • Viral encephalitis

KEY POINTS

- West Nile Virus (WNV) is the most widely distributed flavivirus and causes multiple viral encephalitis outbreaks in humans in different regions worldwide.
- Nearly half of the WNV convalescent patients are reported to have persistent neurologic sequelae or chronic kidney disease.
- Neither treatment nor vaccines are available for human use; current efforts on drug development have been mostly focused on the inhibitors of virus replication.
- Results from field and animal model studies will provide important new insights onto WNV transmission, host immunity, and viral pathogenesis; the findings will also lead to the development of new strategies to prevent and treat WNV-induced encephalitis.

INTRODUCTION

West Nile virus (WNV), a mosquito-borne, single-stranded, positive-sense flavivirus, has been the leading cause of arboviral encephalitis globally. The virus was originally isolated from Uganda in 1937; later caused epidemic outbreaks in Asia, Europe, and Australia; and was introduced into the United States in 1999.[1] The genome of WNV is approximately 11,000 nucleotides in length, which is translated and processed into 10 proteins: 3 structural proteins (envelope [E], membrane, nucleocapsid) and 7 nonstructural (NS) proteins (NS1, NS2A, NS2B, NS3, NS4A, NS4B, and NS5).[2,3]

Although most human infections are asymptomatic, approximately 20% of the infected individuals become symptomatic and develop acute illness, ranging from systemic flu like illness, such as West Nile fever, to neuroinvasive outcomes.[4] In fewer

Disclosure: This work was supported in part by National Institutes of Health grant R01AI099123 (T.W.).
^a Department of Immunology and Serology, National AIDS Research Institute, G-73, MIDC, Bhosari, Pune, Maharashtra 411026, India; ^b Arbovirus Laboratory, Texas Department of State Health Services, 1100 West 49th Street, Austin, TX 78714, USA; ^c Department of Microbiology & Immunology, University of Texas Medical Branch, Keiller 3.118B, Galveston, TX 77555-0609, USA; ^d Department of Pathology, University of Texas Medical Branch, 301 University Boulevard, Galveston, TX 77555, USA
* Corresponding author. Department of Microbiology & Immunology, University of Texas Medical Branch, Keiller 3.118B, Galveston, TX 77555-0609.
E-mail address: ti1wang@utmb.edu

than 1% of the symptomatic individuals, virus entry into the central nervous system (CNS) results in neuroinvasive manifestations, such as meningitis, encephalitis, poliomyelitis, and death.[5,6] Both older adults and immunocompromised individuals are at a high risk of developing neuroinvasive disease.[7,8] Ocular manifestations including multifocal choroiditis, retinal hemorrhage, chorioretinal lesions, optic neuritis, and vitritis are also known to be associated with WNV infection.[9–13] Up to 50% of convalescent patients with WNV are reported to have persistent neurologic sequelae or chronic kidney disease, which occurs 6 to 12 months after the acute infection.[14–17] Moreover, follow-up clinical studies reported that some convalescent patients and asymptomatic WNV RNA-positive blood donors, continue to have detectable serum or cerebrospinal fluid (CSF) levels of WNV-specific immunoglobulin (Ig)M and IgA for more than 6 months and up to several years after their initial infection.[18] These facts indicate that WNV antigen may persist in the periphery or in the CNS in humans after acute infection. Indeed, the persistence of WNV antigen and RNA in the CNS of an immunocompromised patient[19] and presence of WNV RNA in urine of convalescent patients with WNV neuroinvasive disease after 1 to 7 years[20] present the evidence of chronic infection. Neither treatment nor vaccines are currently available for human use. In this review, we discuss recent findings from studies in field and animal models of WNV infection and provide new insights onto WNV transmission, host immunity, viral pathogenesis, diagnosis, and vaccine development.

TRANSMISSION CYCLE

WNV is primarily maintained in nature by transmission between ornithophilic *Culex* mosquitoes and a variety of bird species (**Fig. 1**). In the United States, the virus has been detected in 65 different species of mosquitoes.[21] However, only a few of *Culex* species have been reported to drive epidemic transmission to humans and other vertebrates and these primary vector species vary by geographic region.[21] Generally, in the western part of the United States, *Culex tarsalis* mosquitoes are the major WNV

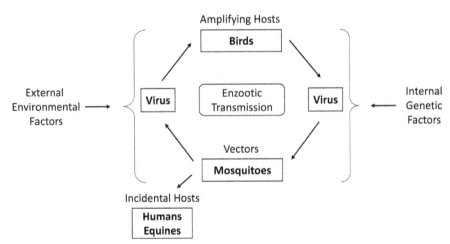

Fig. 1. West Nile virus transmission cycle. The virus is maintained in nature by an enzootic transmission cycle between mosquitoes and avian hosts. Humans and horses are considered incidental or "dead-end" hosts, as they do not generate sufficient viremia to support ongoing transmission. Numerous external environmental factors and internal genetic factors can affect the transmission cycle.

vector species,[22,23] in the eastern states, it is primarily *Culex pipiens*,[24] and in the southeastern states are *Culex quinquefasciatus* and *Culex nigripalpus*.[25–27] Humans and horses are incidental or dead-end hosts, as duration of viremia is brief and not sufficient to infect mosquitoes.[28] Besides mosquito bites, other routes of human infection are blood transfusions,[29] organ transplantation,[30] and breastfeeding,[31] and there is also evidence suggesting potential transmission in utero.[32] Numerous external and internal factors can contribute to the interactions between vector, vertebrate host, and pathogen (see **Fig. 1**). External factors, such as temperature, humidity, precipitation,[33] and landscape structure,[34] can affect transmission cycle of arboviruses between vectors and vertebrate hosts.[35] For example, warmer temperatures tend to increase vector populations, the frequency of blood feeding and oviposition, and the rate of pathogen development in the vector, which results in a shorter extrinsic incubation period.[34] In addition, there is clearly an association between rainfall and abundance of larval habitats, therefore influencing mosquito population size.[36] Many intrinsic factors are also involved in WNV transmission, including vector competence of mosquito species,[28] susceptibility of host species,[37] and the pathogenicity of circulating viral strains.[38]

ANIMAL MODELS

Various experimental animal models have been used to study acute and persistent WNV infection, including monkeys,[39] hamsters,[40] rabbits,[41] and mice.[42] The first well-documented WNV persistence was reported by Pogodina,[39] in nonhuman primates in 1983, in which infectious virus was detected in the CNS tissues and kidneys for up to 5.5 months. Systemic infection in hamsters with wild-type WNV resulted in virus persistence in the brain and chronic viruria along with neuropathological lesions and renal histopathologic changes for up to several months.[40,43,44] Nevertheless, due to regulatory issues and limited availability of reagents, neither animal models are ideal for investigating host immunity to WNV infection. Mice are generally susceptible to WNV infection, easiest to work with, economical, and are most amenable to immunologic manipulation. Following a subcutaneous or intraperitoneal inoculation, the virus induces a brief viremia and eventually invades the CNS. The severity and symptoms of acute WNV infection observed in mice mimic severe cases observed in humans. In addition, WNV infection in mice either by the wild-type strain or an isolate cultured from the urine of a persistently infected hamster shares some similarity and discrepancy in symptoms and tissue tropism with the clinical findings in some convalescent patients with WNV having long-term morbidity, such as chronic kidney diseases or long-term neurologic sequelae.[42,45] Thus, the murine model is an effective in vivo experimental model to investigate viral pathogenesis and the host immunity in humans.

PROTECTIVE HOST IMMUNITY

Studies from animal models suggest that both innate and adaptive responses are involved in host defense against WNV infection. Initially, the signaling pathways of several pathogen recognition receptors, including toll-like receptors (TLRs) 3 and 7 and RIG-I–like receptors (RLRs) are induced by the virus to boost innate immunity and culminate in the synthesis of antiviral cytokines, such as type I interferons (IFNs) and proinflammatory cytokines.[46–49] Type I IFNs and IFN-stimulating genes (ISGs) participate in the control of viral infections and prevent WNV from invading into the brain.[50–53] Recent studies[54,55] have shown that type I and type III (IFN-λ) are implicated in promoting blood brain barrier (BBB) integrity, and decrease WNV entry into the CNS. Next, $\gamma\delta$ T cells, one of the innate immune cells, play a role in the early control of WNV dissemination, mainly through the secretion of IFN-γ[56–58] and regulate adaptive immunity by promoting dendritic cell (DC) maturation and T-cell priming during WNV infection.[59] B cells and specific antibodies are critical in the control of disseminated WNV infection, but are not sufficient to eliminate it from the host[60–63]; whereas the complement system limits WNV replication, in part through its ability to induce a protective antibody response and by priming adaptive immune responses via distinct mechanisms.[64,65] Finally, $\alpha\beta^+$ T cells provide long-lasting protective immunity after WNV infection. CD4$^+$ T cells provide help for antibody responses and sustain WNV-specific CD8$^+$ T-cell responses in the tissues that enable viral clearance.[66] In particular, induction of peripheral T regulatory cells after infection protect against severe WNV disease in immunocompetent animals and humans[67] and are essential for generating a pool of WNV-specific memory T cells.[68] CD8$^+$ T-cell responses are critical in clearing WNV infection from tissues and preventing viral persistence.[69]

VIRAL PATHOGENESIS

Animal model studies have provided important insights into WNV pathogenesis. On probing and feeding on a live host, mosquitoes inoculate high doses of WNV extravascularly (up to 10^6 plaque-forming units) and low doses intravascularly.[70] Mosquito saliva potentiates the virus replication in the host by reducing the antiviral inflammatory environment and increasing immunosuppressive interleukin (IL)-10 levels and thus maintains a reduced antiviral state.[71,72] Initial virus replication occurs at the epidermal site in keratinocytes by inducing a TLR7-dependent innate cytokine responses, which helps to promote Langerhans cell migration from the epidermis and accumulation in the local draining lymph nodes, where the virus is amplified before dissemination to kidney, spleen, and other visceral organs.[73–75]

In the peripheral organs, plausible target cells for infection are DCs, macrophages, and neutrophils.[76,77] Viral replication peaks at approximately day 4 in blood and spleen.[78] Various host (age and immunocompromised status)[79] and viral factors[80,81] could be implicated for virus entry into brain. The mechanism of neuroinvasion is not clearly defined; however, several routs of entry have been proposed: (1) entry through disrupted BBB caused by tumor necrosis factor-α, IL-1β, and macrophage migration inhibitory factor contribute to the disruption of the BBB,[46,54,82] and matrix metalloproteinases-9 (MMP-9)[83,84]; (2) entry through choroid plexus epithelial cells[85]; (3) infecting olfactory neurons and spreading via the olfactory bulb[86]; and (4) Trojan horse mechanism mediated by infected immune cell infiltration into the CNS.[86] Once inside the brain, WNV-induced CNS disease can be caused by neuronal degeneration, a direct result of viral infection, and/or by bystander damage from the immune response to the pathogen, including lymphocyte and microglial cell responses.[87–90]

DIAGNOSIS AND VACCINE DEVELOPMENT

Detection of WNV-specific antibodies and virus in clinical specimens has been used for diagnosis of a WNV infection. IgM antibodies can be detected in serum at least 8 days and up to 45 days after onset of symptoms,[91] allowing for early diagnosis and differentiation between recent and old infections or vaccinations.[92] Thus, IgM antibody capture enzyme-linked immunosorbent assay (MAC-ELISA) is used to detect WNV-specific antibodies in serum or CSF[21] and a positive result from a single acute-phase clinical specimen suggests evidence of recent infection. A significant weakness of this assay is the cross-reactivity among flaviviruses.[93] The plaque reduction neutralization test provides a confirmatory test for specific diagnosis of WNV infection, although the assay is complex and laborious and requires viable virus isolates under BSL-3 research laboratories.[94] WNV diagnosis also can be determined by virus isolation or detection of viral RNA from serum, CSF, or tissue specimens collected early in the course of illness. These methods have limited utility, because viremia titers are typically low and do not last very long and are often absent by the time neurologic symptoms develop.[95] Alternatively, nucleic acid testing involves amplification of WNV RNA, and is considered more sensitive compared with virus isolation.[94]

There are no licensed human WNV vaccines, but there are multiple equine vaccines, including formalin-inactivated virus, recombinant canarypox, DNA, and chimeric YF-WNV. The latter vaccine was withdrawn from the market in 2010 because of adverse events. Multiple candidate vaccines exist for humans, including inactivated, recombinant live virus, chimeric virus (ChimeriVax-WN), DNA, and recombinant subunit vaccines. Currently, none of these vaccine candidates have progressed beyond clinical evaluation. Although the live vaccine candidates induced high humoral and cell-mediated immune response similar to that obtained with wild-type WNV,[96] vaccination has raised some safety concerns in susceptible individuals.[92] Recombinant subunit vaccines are constructed from the E gene of WNV NY99 strain; however, the major drawback of these subunit vaccines is the high number of doses required to elicit effective protective immunity.[97–99] The development of safe and effective vaccines against WNV remains as a high priority.

SUMMARY

WNV is the most widely distributed flavivirus and causes multiple viral encephalitis outbreaks in humans in different regions worldwide. Nearly half of the convalescent patients with WNV are reported to have persistent neurologic sequelae or chronic kidney disease. Neither treatment nor vaccines are available for human use. Current efforts on drug development have mostly been focused on the inhibitors of virus replication. Results from field and animal model studies will provide important new insights onto WNV transmission, host immunity, and viral pathogenesis. The findings also will lead the development of new strategies to prevent and treat WNV-induced encephalitis.

REFERENCES

1. Nash D, Mostashari F, Fine A, et al. The outbreak of West Nile virus infection in the New York City area in 1999. N Engl J Med 2001;344(24):1807–14.
2. Anderson JF, Andreadis TG, Vossbrinck CR, et al. Isolation of West Nile virus from mosquitoes, crows, and a Cooper's hawk in Connecticut. Science 1999; 286(5448):2331–3.
3. Lanciotti RS, Roehrig JT, Deubel V, et al. Origin of the West Nile virus responsible for an outbreak of encephalitis in the northeastern United States. Science 1999; 286(5448):2333–7.
4. Mostashari F, Bunning ML, Kitsutani PT, et al. Epidemic West Nile encephalitis, New York, 1999: results of a household-based seroepidemiological survey. Lancet 2001;358(9278):261–4.
5. Gubler DJ. The continuing spread of West Nile virus in the western hemisphere. Clin Infect Dis 2007;45(8):1039–46.
6. Kramer LD, Styer LM, Ebel GD. A global perspective on the epidemiology of West Nile virus. Annu Rev Entomol 2008;53:61–81.

7. O'Leary DR, Marfin AA, Montgomery SP, et al. The epidemic of West Nile virus in the United States, 2002. Vector Borne Zoonotic Dis 2004;4(1):61–70.

8. Murray K, Baraniuk S, Resnick M, et al. Risk factors for encephalitis and death from West Nile virus infection. Epidemiol Infect 2006;134(6):1325–32.

9. Vandenbelt S, Shaikh S, Capone A Jr, et al. Multifocal choroiditis associated with West Nile virus encephalitis. Retina 2003;23(1):97–9.

10. Hershberger VS, Augsburger JJ, Hutchins RK, et al. Chorioretinal lesions in nonfatal cases of West Nile virus infection. Ophthalmology 2003;110(9):1732–6.

11. Adelman RA, Membreno JH, Afshari NA, et al. West Nile virus chorioretinitis. Retina 2003;23(1):100–1.

12. Gilad R, Lampl Y, Sadeh M, et al. Optic neuritis complicating West Nile virus meningitis in a young adult. Infection 2003;31(1):55–6.

13. Bains HS, Jampol LM, Caughron MC, et al. Vitritis and chorioretinitis in a patient with West Nile virus infection. Arch Ophthalmol 2003;121(2):205–7.

14. Carson PJ, Konewko P, Wold KS, et al. Long-term clinical and neuropsychological outcomes of West Nile virus infection. Clin Infect Dis 2006;43(6):723–30.

15. Cook RL, Xu X, Yablonsky EJ, et al. Demographic and clinical factors associated with persistent symptoms after West Nile virus infection. Am J Trop Med Hyg 2010;83(5):1133–6.

16. Sadek JR, Pergam SA, Harrington JA, et al. Persistent neuropsychological impairment associated with West Nile virus infection. J Clin Exp Neuropsychol 2010; 32(1):81–7.

17. Nolan MS, Podoll AS, Hause AM, et al. Prevalence of chronic kidney disease and progression of disease over time among patients enrolled in the Houston West Nile virus cohort. PLoS One 2012;7(7):e40374.

18. Busch MP, Kleinman SH, Tobler LH, et al. Virus and antibody dynamics in acute West Nile virus infection. J Infect Dis 2008;198(7):984–93.

19. Penn RG, Guarner J, Sejvar JJ, et al. Persistent neuroinvasive West Nile virus infection in an immunocompromised patient. Clin Infect Dis 2006;42(5):680–3.

20. Murray K, Walker C, Herrington E, et al. Persistent infection with West Nile virus years after initial infection. J Infect Dis 2010;201(1):2–4.

21. Petersen LR, Brault AC, Nasci RS. West Nile virus: review of the literature. JAMA 2013;310(3):308–15.

22. Bolling BG, Moore CG, Anderson SL, et al. Entomological studies along the Colorado Front Range during a period of intense West Nile virus activity. J Am Mosq Control Assoc 2007;23(1):37–46.

23. Goddard LB, Roth AE, Reisen WK, et al. Vector competence of California mosquitoes for West Nile virus. Emerg Infect Dis 2002;8(12):1385–91.

24. Andreadis TG, Anderson JF, Vossbrinck CR, et al. Epidemiology of West Nile virus in Connecticut: a five-year analysis of mosquito data 1999-2003. Vector Borne Zoonotic Dis 2004;4(4):360–78.

25. Godsey MS Jr, Blackmore MS, Panella NA, et al. West Nile virus epizootiology in the southeastern United States, 2001. Vector Borne Zoonotic Dis 2005;5(1):82–9.

26. Godsey MS Jr, King RJ, Burkhalter K, et al. Ecology of potential West Nile virus vectors in Southeastern Louisiana: enzootic transmission in the relative absence of Culex quinquefasciatus. Am J Trop Med Hyg 2013;88(5):986–96.

27. Rutledge CR, Day JF, Lord CC, et al. West Nile virus infection rates in Culex nigripalpus (Diptera: Culicidae) do not reflect transmission rates in Florida. J Med Entomol 2003;40(3):253–8.

28. Ciota AT, Kramer LD. Vector-virus interactions and transmission dynamics of West Nile virus. Viruses 2013;5(12):3021–47.

29. Stramer SL, Fang CT, Foster GA, et al. West Nile virus among blood donors in the United States, 2003 and 2004. N Engl J Med 2005;353(5):451–9.
30. Mezochow AK, Henry R, Blumberg EA, et al. Transfusion transmitted infections in solid organ transplantation. Am J Transplant 2015;15(2):547–54.
31. Kramer LD, Li J, Shi PY. West Nile virus. Lancet Neurol 2007;6(2):171–81.
32. O'Leary DR, Kuhn S, Kniss KL, et al. Birth outcomes following West Nile Virus infection of pregnant women in the United States: 2003-2004. Pediatrics 2006; 117(3):e537–45.
33. Moore CG. Interdisciplinary research in the ecology of vector-borne diseases: opportunities and needs. J Vector Ecol 2008;33(2):218–24.
34. Reisen WK. Landscape epidemiology of vector-borne diseases. Annu Rev Entomol 2010;55:461–83.
35. Gould EA, Higgs S. Impact of climate change and other factors on emerging arbovirus diseases. Trans R Soc Trop Med Hyg 2009;103(2):109–21.
36. Reisen WK, Cayan D, Tyree M, et al. Impact of climate variation on mosquito abundance in California. J Vector Ecol 2008;33(1):89–98.
37. Brault AC. Changing patterns of West Nile virus transmission: altered vector competence and host susceptibility. Vet Res 2009;40(2):43.
38. Kilpatrick AM, Meola MA, Moudy RM, et al. Temperature, viral genetics, and the transmission of West Nile virus by *Culex pipiens* mosquitoes. PLoS Pathog 2008; 4(6):e1000092.
39. Pogodina VV, Frolova MP, Malenko GV, et al. Study on West Nile virus persistence in monkeys. Arch Virol 1983;75(1–2):71–86.
40. Tesh RB, Siirin M, Guzman H, et al. Persistent West Nile virus infection in the golden hamster: studies on its mechanism and possible implications for other flavivirus infections. J Infect Dis 2005;192(2):287–95.
41. Suen WW, Uddin MJ, Wang W, et al. Experimental West Nile Virus infection in rabbits: an alternative model for studying induction of disease and virus control. Pathogens 2015;4(3):529–58.
42. Appler KK, Brown AN, Stewart BS, et al. Persistence of West Nile virus in the central nervous system and periphery of mice. PLoS One 2010;5(5):e10649.
43. Siddharthan V, Wang H, Motter NE, et al. Persistent West Nile virus associated with a neurological sequela in hamsters identified by motor unit number estimation. J Virol 2009;83(9):4251–61.
44. Tesh RB, Xiao SY. Persistence of West Nile virus infection in vertebrates. In: Diamond MS, editor. West Nile encephalitis virus infection viral pathogenesis and host response. New York: Springer; 2009. p. 361–77.
45. Saxena V, Xie G, Li B, et al. A hamster-derived West Nile virus isolate induces persistent renal infection in mice. PLoS Negl Trop Dis 2013;7(6):e2275.
46. Wang T, Town T, Alexopoulou L, et al. Toll-like receptor 3 mediates West Nile virus entry into the brain causing lethal encephalitis. Nat Med 2004;10(12):1366–73.
47. Errett JS, Suthar MS, McMillan A, et al. The essential, nonredundant roles of RIG-I and MDA5 in detecting and controlling West Nile virus infection. J Virol 2013; 87(21):11416–25.
48. Town T, Bai F, Wang T, et al. Toll-like receptor 7 mitigates lethal West Nile encephalitis via interleukin 23-dependent immune cell infiltration and homing. Immunity 2009;30(2):242–53.
49. Fredericksen BL, Keller BC, Fornek J, et al. Establishment and maintenance of the innate antiviral response to West Nile Virus involves both RIG-I and MDA5 signaling through IPS-1. J Virol 2008;82(2):609–16.

50. Katze MG, He Y, Gale M Jr. Viruses and interferon: a fight for supremacy. Nat Rev Immunol 2002;2(9):675–87.

51. Samuel MA, Diamond MS. Alpha/beta interferon protects against lethal West Nile virus infection by restricting cellular tropism and enhancing neuronal survival. J Virol 2005;79(21):13350–61.

52. Lazear HM, Pinto AK, Vogt MR, et al. Beta interferon controls West Nile virus infection and pathogenesis in mice. J Virol 2011;85(14):7186–94.

53. Thackray LB, Shrestha B, Richner JM, et al. Interferon regulatory factor 5-dependent immune responses in the draining lymph node protect against West Nile virus infection. J Virol 2014;88(19):11007–21.

54. Daniels BP, Holman DW, Cruz-Orengo L, et al. Viral pathogen-associated molecular patterns regulate blood-brain barrier integrity via competing innate cytokine signals. MBio 2014;5(5):e01476–514.

55. Lazear HM, Daniels BP, Pinto AK, et al. Interferon-lambda restricts West Nile virus neuroinvasion by tightening the blood-brain barrier. Sci Transl Med 2015;7(284): 284ra259.

56. Wang T, Scully E, Yin Z, et al. IFN-gamma-producing gammadelta T cells help control murine West Nile virus infection. J Immunol 2003;171(5):2524–31.

57. Shrestha B, Wang T, Samuel MA, et al. Gamma interferon plays a crucial early antiviral role in protection against West Nile virus infection. J Virol 2006;80(11): 5338–48.

58. Welte T, Lamb J, Anderson JF, et al. Role of two distinct gammadelta T cell subsets during West Nile virus infection. FEMS Immunol Med Microbiol 2008;53(2): 275–83.

59. Fang H, Welte T, Zheng X, et al. Gammadelta T cells promote the maturation of dendritic cells during West Nile virus infection. FEMS Immunol Med Microbiol 2010;59(1):71–80.

60. Diamond MS, Shrestha B, Marri A, et al. B cells and antibody play critical roles in the immediate defense of disseminated infection by West Nile encephalitis virus. J Virol 2003;77(4):2578–86.

61. Diamond MS, Shrestha B, Mehlhop E, et al. Innate and adaptive immune responses determine protection against disseminated infection by West Nile encephalitis virus. Viral Immunol 2003;16(3):259–78.

62. Diamond MS, Sitati EM, Friend LD, et al. A critical role for induced IgM in the protection against West Nile virus infection. J Exp Med 2003;198(12):1853–62.

63. Roehrig JT, Staudinger LA, Hunt AR, et al. Antibody prophylaxis and therapy for flavivirus encephalitis infections. Ann N Y Acad Sci 2001;951:286–97.

64. Mehlhop E, Diamond MS. Protective immune responses against West Nile virus are primed by distinct complement activation pathways. J Exp Med 2006; 203(5):1371–81.

65. Mehlhop E, Whitby K, Oliphant T, et al. Complement activation is required for induction of a protective antibody response against West Nile virus infection. J Virol 2005;79(12):7466–77.

66. Sitati EM, Diamond MS. CD4+ T-cell responses are required for clearance of West Nile virus from the central nervous system. J Virol 2006;80(24):12060–9.

67. Lanteri MC, O'Brien KM, Purtha WE, et al. Tregs control the development of symptomatic West Nile virus infection in humans and mice. J Clin Invest 2009;119(11): 3266–77.

68. Graham JB, Da Costa A, Lund JM. Regulatory T cells shape the resident memory T cell response to virus infection in the tissues. J Immunol 2014;192(2):683–90.

69. Shrestha B, Diamond MS. Role of CD8+ T cells in control of West Nile virus infection. J Virol 2004;78(15):8312–21.

70. Styer LM, Kent KA, Albright RG, et al. Mosquitoes inoculate high doses of West Nile virus as they probe and feed on live hosts. PLoS Pathog 2007;3(9):1262–70.

71. Moser LA, Lim PY, Styer LM, et al. Parameters of mosquito-enhanced West Nile Virus infection. J Virol 2016;90(1):292–9.

72. Schneider BS, Soong L, Girard YA, et al. Potentiation of West Nile encephalitis by mosquito feeding. Viral Immunol 2006;19(1):74–82.

73. Byrne SN, Halliday GM, Johnston LJ, et al. Interleukin-1beta but not tumor necrosis factor is involved in West Nile virus-induced Langerhans cell migration from the skin in C57BL/6 mice. J Invest Dermatol 2001;117(3):702–9.

74. Lim PY, Behr MJ, Chadwick CM, et al. Keratinocytes are cell targets of West Nile virus in vivo. J Virol 2011;85(10):5197–201.

75. Welte T, Reagan K, Fang H, et al. Toll-like receptor 7-induced immune response to cutaneous West Nile virus infection. J Gen Virol 2009;90(Pt 11):2660–8.

76. Bai F, Kong KF, Dai J, et al. A paradoxical role for neutrophils in the pathogenesis of West Nile virus. J Infect Dis 2010;202(12):1804–12.

77. Ben-Nathan D, Huitinga I, Lustig S, et al. West Nile virus neuroinvasion and encephalitis induced by macrophage depletion in mice. Arch Virol 1996;141(3–4):459–69.

78. Suthar MS, Diamond MS, Gale M Jr. West Nile virus infection and immunity. Nat Rev Microbiol 2013;11(2):115–28.

79. Sejvar JJ. Clinical manifestations and outcomes of West Nile virus infection. Viruses 2014;6(2):606–23.

80. Beasley DW, Li L, Suderman MT, et al. Mouse neuroinvasive phenotype of West Nile virus strains varies depending upon virus genotype. Virology 2002;296(1):17–23.

81. Beasley DW, Whiteman MC, Zhang S, et al. Envelope protein glycosylation status influences mouse neuroinvasion phenotype of genetic lineage 1 West Nile virus strains. J Virol 2005;79(13):8339–47.

82. Arjona A, Foellmer HG, Town T, et al. Abrogation of macrophage migration inhibitory factor decreases West Nile virus lethality by limiting viral neuroinvasion. J Clin Invest 2007;117(10):3059–66.

83. Wang P, Dai J, Bai F, et al. Matrix metalloproteinase 9 facilitates West Nile virus entry into the brain. J Virol 2008;82(18):8978–85.

84. Verma S, Kumar M, Gurjav U, et al. Reversal of West Nile virus-induced blood-brain barrier disruption and tight junction proteins degradation by matrix metalloproteinases inhibitor. Virology 2010;397(1):130–8.

85. Samuel MA, Wang H, Siddharthan V, et al. Axonal transport mediates West Nile virus entry into the central nervous system and induces acute flaccid paralysis. Proc Natl Acad Sci U S A 2007;104(43):17140–5.

86. Samuel MA, Diamond MS. Pathogenesis of West Nile Virus infection: a balance between virulence, innate and adaptive immunity, and viral evasion. J Virol 2006;80(19):9349–60.

87. Sampson BA, Armbrustmacher V. West Nile encephalitis: the neuropathology of four fatalities. Ann N Y Acad Sci 2001;951:172–8.

88. Shrestha B, Gottlieb D, Diamond MS. Infection and injury of neurons by West Nile encephalitis virus. J Virol 2003;77(24):13203–13.

89. Wang Y, Lobigs M, Lee E, et al. CD8+ T cells mediate recovery and immunopathology in West Nile virus encephalitis. J Virol 2003;77(24):13323–34.

90. Xiao SY, Guzman H, Zhang H, et al. West Nile virus infection in the golden hamster (*Mesocricetus auratus*): a model for West Nile encephalitis. Emerg Infect Dis 2001;7(4):714–21.
91. Martin DA, Muth DA, Brown T, et al. Standardization of immunoglobulin M capture enzyme-linked immunosorbent assays for routine diagnosis of arboviral infections. J Clin Microbiol 2000;38(5):1823–6.
92. Dauphin G, Zientara S. West Nile virus: recent trends in diagnosis and vaccine development. Vaccine 2007;25(30):5563–76.
93. Roehrig JT. West Nile virus in the United States - a historical perspective. Viruses 2013;5(12):3088–108.
94. De Filette M, Ulbert S, Diamond M, et al. Recent progress in West Nile virus diagnosis and vaccination. Vet Res 2012;43:16.
95. Hayes EB, Komar N, Nasci RS, et al. Epidemiology and transmission dynamics of West Nile virus disease. Emerg Infect Dis 2005;11(8):1167–73.
96. Monath TP. Prospects for development of a vaccine against the West Nile virus. Ann N Y Acad Sci 2001;951:1–12.
97. Ledizet M, Kar K, Foellmer HG, et al. A recombinant envelope protein vaccine against West Nile virus. Vaccine 2005;23(30):3915–24.
98. Wang T, Anderson JF, Magnarelli LA, et al. Immunization of mice against West Nile virus with recombinant envelope protein. J Immunol 2001;167(9):5273–7.
99. Qiao M, Ashok M, Bernard KA, et al. Induction of sterilizing immunity against West Nile Virus (WNV), by immunization with WNV-like particles produced in insect cells. J Infect Dis 2004;190(12):2104–8.

Zika Virus

Ryan F. Relich, PhD, D(ABMM), MLS(ASCP)SM[a],*,
Michael Loeffelholz, PhD, D(ABMM)[b]

KEYWORDS

- Arbovirus • Autochthonous • Birth defects • Flavivirus • *Flaviviridae*
- Guillain-Barré syndrome • Microcephaply

KEY POINTS

- Before its emergence in Brazil in 2015, Zika virus was not thought to be endemically transmitted in the Americas. Since then, it has spread across South America and into North America, including the Caribbean and, recently, the United States.
- Zika virus is most commonly transmitted by mosquitoes; however, horizontal and vertical transmission in humans is well documented.
- Zika fever presents with similar symptoms to other arboviral infections, so both molecular and serologic testing are required to distinguish it from similar diseases.
- Birth defects and serious neurologic sequelae have been recorded in association with Zika virus infection.
- Continued epidemiologic monitoring as well as basic research into the biology, pathogenesis, and immunology of Zika virus and Zika fever is needed to develop effective countermeasures and vaccines.

INTRODUCTION

Before 2015, Zika virus (ZIKV), a once obscure mosquito-borne virus, was responsible for sporadic outbreaks of acute febrile illness in parts of the Eastern Hemisphere. In early 2015, a cluster of dengue fever–like illnesses characterized by fever, maculopapular rash, arthralgia/myalgias, and conjunctivitis was reported in the Brazilian city of Camaçari, in the state of Bahia.[1] ZIKV RNA was detected by polymerase chain reaction (PCR) in serum specimens from 7/24 (29.2%) patients who received care at Santa Helena Hospital. By December of that year, between 440,000 and 1,300,000 human ZIKV infections were estimated to have occurred.[2] As of September 2016, widespread

Disclosures: The authors have no potential conflicts of interest to report.
[a] Department of Pathology and Laboratory Medicine, Indiana University School of Medicine, 350 West 11th Street, Suite 6027, Indianapolis, IN 46202, USA; [b] Clinical Microbiology Laboratory, Department of Pathology, University of Texas Medical Branch, 301 University Boulevard, Galveston, TX 77555-0740, USA
* Corresponding author.
E-mail address: rrelich@iupui.edu

autochthonous transmission of ZIKV has been documented in nearly every country in the Western Hemisphere, demonstrating the rapidity with which emerging infectious diseases can spread in immunologically naïve populations, especially if competent vectors and potential reservoir species are present in disease-endemic regions.

ZIKV was discovered in April 1947 as a result of investigating the cause of fever in a sentinel rhesus monkey, animal number 766, that was placed in the Zika forest of Uganda as part of a yellow fever research mission sponsored by the Rockefeller Foundation.[3] ZIKV was ultimately isolated from the brains of Swiss albino mice that were intracerebrally inoculated with serum collected from rhesus 766. Nine months later, in January 1948, ZIKV was again isolated, only this time from brain tissue of mice intracerebrally inoculated with clarified homogenates of *Aedes africanus* mosquitoes collected from the Zika forest.[3] It was not until 1954 that the first human cases of Zika fever were documented. Briefly, 3 Nigerian patients, a 30-year-old man (patient 1), a 24-year-old man (patient 2), and a 10-year-old girl (patient 3), presented with mild pyrexia, headache, and other symptoms. ZIKV was later isolated from the serum of patient 3 via intracerebral inoculation of mice, and anti-ZIKV antibodies were detected in the sera of patients 1 and 2.[4] Since then, ZIKV serosurveys have identified human and animal ZIKV exposures throughout Africa and Asia, demonstrating the extensive endemicity of this virus. Results of these studies should be interpreted with caution, however, because serologic tests for ZIKV are prone to cross-reactivity with antibodies generated in response to related viruses, including Spondweni virus, dengue virus (DENV), and others.[5] In 2007, an outbreak of Zika fever on Yap Island in the Western Pacific marked the first time that ZIKV was detected outside of Africa and mainland Asia.[6] In the following years, additional outbreaks across the Pacific region were documented, including a very large epidemic spanning all of the archipelagoes of French Polynesia, and later, in New Caledonia, Cook Islands, Easter Island, Fiji, Vanuatu, and others.[5,7,8] Ultimately, phylogenetic and phylogeographic data conclude that the current epidemic in the Western Hemisphere resulted from the introduction of ZIKV from French Polynesia by way of Easter Island into mainland South America.[9]

To date, little is understood about the dynamics of ZIKV infection, and new modes of transmission, including sexual intercourse, as well as the appearance of severe complications, including birth defects and neurologic diseases, have only recently been described. Newly established animal and cell culture models of ZIKV infection have provided some insight into the pathogenicity of ZIKV, but these systems are still in their infancy and have yet to reproducibly recapitulate the more severe complications observed in human infections. The paucity of information regarding the myriad aspects of Zika fever pathophysiology and the long-term consequences of pregnancy-associated ZIKV infections have prompted a multinational effort to develop targeted therapeutics, effective vector control programs, and vaccines to protect vulnerable populations. Because of the nearly daily release of new publications concerning information about ZIKV and Zika fever, it is impossible to review the entire body of current knowledge; however, the authors have attempted to summarize salient points regarding the epidemiology, basic biology, pathophysiology, diagnosis, treatment, and prevention of ZIKV infection.

EPIDEMIOLOGY

Between 1947 and 2014, ZIKV was associated with sporadic epidemics in parts of Africa, Southeast Asia, and Oceania. The most extensive epidemic during this time period occurred in French Polynesia in 2013; approximately 30,000 cases were suspected, affecting 11.5% of the total population. This epidemic marked the first occasion of widespread arboviral disease not associated with DENV on the archipelagoes of French Polynesia.[1,9] In February 2014 on the South Pacific island nation of New Caledonia, a ZIKV outbreak was declared, which stemmed from travel-associated cases in people who had visited French Polynesia in the latter part of 2013. By late August 2014, approximately 1400 cases were reported. Subsequent outbreaks on the Cook Islands and Easter Island also occurred in 2014; however, in both outbreaks, the total number of cases was less than 1000.[10,11] In 2015, small outbreaks of Zika fever were reported from Vanuatu, the Solomon Islands, Samoa, and Fiji. In each of the aforementioned outbreaks, exported cases of ZIKV infection were reported in several countries, including Australia, England, Italy, Japan, New Zealand, and the United States, to name a few.[9]

Since its discovery until 2015, virtually all cases of Zika fever diagnosed in the Western Hemisphere were in patients who had recently traveled to regions of the Eastern Hemisphere experiencing ongoing ZIKV transmission. However, a recent report by Lednicky and colleagues[12] describes locally acquired Zika fever among 3 school children from 3 different rural areas of Haiti in December 2014. Briefly, ZIKV was isolated from the blood of these patients during an investigation of DENV and chikungunya virus (CHIKV) infections in Haiti. Clinical samples that were negative for both DENV and CHIKV were further screened by cell culture for the presence of agents likely to be associated with DENV- and CHIKV-like illness in the study population. The findings of this investigation demonstrated the existence of autochthonous ZIKV transmission in the Western Hemisphere before its detection in Brazil the following year.

In late 2014, numerous cases of an exanthematous illness were reported from several regions in Brazil. Later, serologic and molecular testing implicated ZIKV in many, but not all, cases. In 2015, autochthonous transmission of ZIKV in Brazil was confirmed and, since then, ZIKV has spread extensively throughout South America, Central America, the Caribbean, and Mexico. During the summer of 2016, the Florida State Department of Health identified 2 areas of local ZIKV transmission in Miami-Dade County, a finding that added the Unites States to the list of Western countries reporting endemic transmission. In November 2016, the Texas Department of State Health Services reported a case of mosquito-transmitted ZIKV infection in Brownsville, a city of over 420,000 residents located in the southernmost tip of Texas, marking the second geographic region in the U.S. affected by autochthonous ZIKV transmission. As of February 6, 2017, 220 cases of locally acquired, mosquito-transmitted ZIKV infection have been reported and, overall, 4,973 cases, including locally acquired, travel-associated, and 1 case resulting from a laboratory exposure, have been reported in the U.S. Of these cases, 41 have been linked to sexual transmission, and Guillain-Barré syndrome has been documented in 13.[13]

Evidence of ZIKV exposure in both humans and animals has been documented in tropical regions in the Eastern Hemisphere between 1947 and now by way of seroepidemiological surveys, virus isolation, and molecular methods. Data generated by many of these studies suggest that, like other flaviviruses, including yellow fever virus (YFV), ZIKV is maintained in nature by cycling between nonhuman primates or other animal species and competent mosquito vectors or by human-mosquito-human transmission cycles. The latter cycle is thought to be responsible for sustaining ZIKV endemicity in parts of the world where nonhuman primates are not found, such as on Yap Island.[9,14] Detection of ZIKV antibodies in various animal species, including nonhuman primates, sheep, bats, wildebeests, and rodents, suggests that ZIKV can infect and illicit immunologic responses across a broad array of mammalian taxa.[15–18] However, the roles of nonprimate animal species in the maintenance of ZIKV in nature has yet to be entirely demonstrated.[9]

Arthropod Vectors

Mosquitoes are the principal vectors of ZIKV transmission, and several strains of the virus have been isolated from a variety of mosquito species, including *Aedes* spp, *Culex perfuscus*, *Eretmapodites* spp, and *Mansonia* spp from sites across Africa, Asia, the South Pacific and, most recently, the Americas.[9,19] In many outbreaks, the major vector of ZIKV transmission has been either presumed or demonstrated to be one or more *Aedes* spp. In the 2007 ZIKV outbreak on Yap Island, *Aedes hensilli* was presumed to be the major vector of the virus based on the abundance of this species and previous evidence that implicated it in the transmission of DENV on the island.[20] *Aedes albopictus*, the Asian tiger mosquito, has also been linked to ZIKV transmission. Its role as a vector was revealed during concurrent epidemics of chikungunya, dengue, and Zika fevers in Gabon in 2007.[21] In this epidemic, ZIKV RNA was detected in 2 *A albopictus* pools collected in the Gabonese capital city of Libreville by PCR assays targeting the NS5 gene. Later, in the French Polynesian ZIKV outbreak spanning 2013 to 2014, *Aedes polynesiensis*, the Polynesian tiger mosquito, was thought to be involved in transmission, along with *Aedes aegypti*, but a causal link to the former was never determined.[9]

Recently, direct evidence implicating *A aegypti*, the yellow fever mosquito, in ZIKV transmission in North America was published.[19] Because of the pervasiveness of this mosquito in Zika-endemic regions, its role in the transmission of several other arboviruses, and experimental confirmation of its competence as a vector of several strains of ZIKV, it is regarded as the most significant vector of ZIKV. The role of other mosquito species in the transmission of ZIKV is currently a hot topic of research among numerous laboratories throughout the world, and numerous species have been experimentally demonstrated to be susceptible to ZIKV infection. However, in the absence of data demonstrating the capability of a mosquito species to transmit an infectious agent to a susceptible host, it should be noted that detection of ZIKV RNA or infectious ZIKV alone from mosquitoes is insufficient to implicate them as vectors. For a semi-comprehensive list of mosquito species from which ZIKV has been isolated, please see ref.[9]

Person-to-Person Transmission

Horizontal and vertical transmission of ZIKV has been documented in humans. Unprotected sexual intercourse with both infected male and female partners has resulted in sexually acquired Zika fever cases. The first reported instance of sexual transmission of ZIKV was in 2008 in the wife of a 36-year-old male American scientist. The scientist, who, before developing symptoms of Zika fever, lived and worked in the Senegalese village of Bandafassi. Six days after returning to his home in Colorado, the male patient became symptomatic and, 4 days later, his wife developed similar symptoms. Virological testing, including attempts at virus isolation in cell culture and intracerebral inoculation of suckling mice, as well as molecular tests for arboviruses, failed to identify an etiologic agent. Testing of convalescent-phase serum by hemagglutination inhibition, virus neutralization, and complement fixation ultimately identified ZIKV as the most likely culprit.[22] Numerous cases of male-to-female transmission have been reported during the ongoing epidemic in the Americas.

In late August 2016, a nonpregnant woman in her mid twenties who had recently traveled to a region with active ZIKV transmission became symptomatic (headache, abdominal cramping, fever, fatigue, rash, myalgia, arthralgia, and so forth) within

24 hours of arriving to New York City. On the third day of her illness, she presented for medical care, during which time specimens were collected and submitted to the New York City Department of Health and Mental Hygiene (DOHMH) Public Health Laboratory for testing; ZIKV RNA was detected in both her serum and urine. During her assessment, the patient reported that she had a single unprotected sexual encounter with her male partner following her arrival to New York City. Seven days after sexual intercourse, her male partner developed symptoms and subsequently received treatment on day 3 of his illness; ZIKV RNA was detected from his urine but not serum. The male patient denied travel outside of the United States during the entire year before his illness and admitted to having unprotected vaginal intercourse with the female patient on day 0 of her illness. An investigation conducted by the DOHMH concluded that female-to-male horizontal transmission had occurred through vaginal intercourse.[23]

Numerous cases of vertical ZIKV transmission have been reported during the current and past epidemics. However, the severity of congenital infections, ultimately leading to severe birth defects, was not apparent until recently. Coincident with the emergence of ZIKV infection in Brazil in 2015, reports of microcephalic infants being born to mothers who had been infected with ZIKV during pregnancy have surfaced, leading to the hypothetical possibility of an association between the two.[24] Although a relationship between ZIKV infection of pregnant mothers and development of microcephaly and other congenital defects has since been established, factors influencing fetal predisposition for development of birth defects in the context of a ZIKV-infected mother is poorly understood.

Transfusion-based Transmission

The first probable human case of blood transfusion-transmitted ZIKV infection was reported to have occurred in Brazil in July 2016. Shortly after blood donation, the donor experienced symptoms consistent with Zika fever and voluntarily notified the blood donation center of his illness. Unfortunately, the detection of ZIKV in the patient's donated blood came after fractionation of the blood unit and inclusion of the sick donor's platelet concentrate in a pooled platelet unit. The contaminated platelet pool was subsequently transfused into a 55-year-old male liver transplant recipient. Infectious ZIKV and ZIKV nucleic acids were detected in clinical specimens obtained from the recipient 4 days after receiving the platelet transfusion, although the transfusion recipient never became symptomatic.[25] Although no known transfusion-transmitted ZIKV infections have yet been reported in the United States, on August 26, 2016, the US Food and Drug Administration (FDA) revised its guidance regarding ZIKV screening of the US blood supply to include all donated units, and any units shown to be positive for ZIKV nucleic acids are to be removed from the blood supply.[13]

VIROLOGY

ZIKV and its closest relative Spondweni virus comprise the Spondweni virus group within the genus Flavivirus, family Flaviviridae. Currently, there are 2 recognized lineages of ZIKV, African and Asian; the currently circulating strains in the Western Hemisphere appear to be derivatives of the latter. ZIKV particles, like other flaviviruses, are enveloped and spherical and measure approximately 50 nm in diameter (**Fig. 1**). Embedded in the lipid bilayer envelope of mature particles are 180 copies each of the membrane glycoprotein (M) and the envelope glycoprotein (E) that are arranged in an icosahedron-like symmetry.[26] With the exception of approximately 10 amino-acid residues surrounding the Asn^{154} glycosylation site of each envelope glycoprotein,

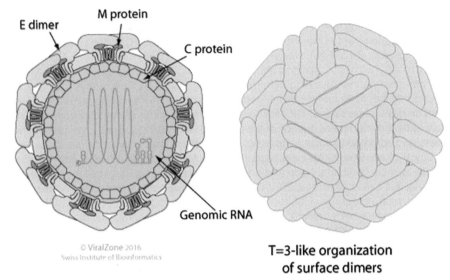

E dimer

M protein

C protein

© ViralZone 2016
Swiss Institute of Bioinformatics

Genomic RNA

T=3-like organization
of surface dimers

Fig. 1. Cartoon of ZIKV showing the enveloped and roughly spherical nature of the virus. Left, in cross-section, the single-stranded, positive-sense RNA genome, the capsid, and the envelope and its associated protein components are shown. Right, the proteins located on the surface (E and M) of a mature, intact particle are arranged in an icosahedron-like symmetry. (Used with permission from Swiss Institute of Bioinformatics, ViralZone [http://viralzone.expasy.org]).

the structure of mature ZIKV is similar to that of other flaviviruses, including DENV and West Nile virus (WNV).[26] Numerous copies of the capsid protein (C) encapsidate the viral genome, which consists of a monopartite, positive-sense, single-stranded RNA molecule measuring approximately 10.8 kb in length. The genome consists of a single open reading frame that encodes 3 structural (capsid protein C [C], membrane glycoprotein precursor M [prM], and envelope protein E [E]) and 7 nonstructural (NS1, NS2A, NS2B, NS3, NS4A, NS4B, and NS5) proteins.[26]

The ZIKV infectious cycle (**Fig. 2**) begins with attachment of virions to the cytoplasmic membrane of susceptible cells, a process mediated by interactions between the viral E protein and one or more host cell receptors, including dendritic cell-specific intercellular adhesion molecule-3-grabbing non-integrin and members of the transmembrane immunoglobulin and mucin domain and Tyro-3, Axl, and Mer families of host cell receptors.[27,28] Virions are next internalized by micropinocytosis, and viral nucleocapsids are eventually released into the cytoplasm following fusion of the viral envelope and the endosomal membrane, a process mediated by the viral E protein following lowering of the endosomal pH. Translation of the viral genome occurs within the cytoplasm, and cotranslational and posttranslational cleavage of the resulting polyprotein into individual proteins is effected by cellular and viral proteases.[9,28,29] Following genome replication and particle assembly within endoplasmic reticulum membrane spherules, particles undergo maturation within the trans-Golgi network. Conformational changes of viral glycoproteins, cleavage of the prM protein into the M protein and pr peptide, and exposure of the E protein fusion domain prime nascent particles for infection of host cells.[30] Egressing transport vesicles are trafficked to the cytoplasmic membrane and, upon fusion of vesicle and cytoplasmic membranes, viral progeny are released from the cell. Like with other viruses, the

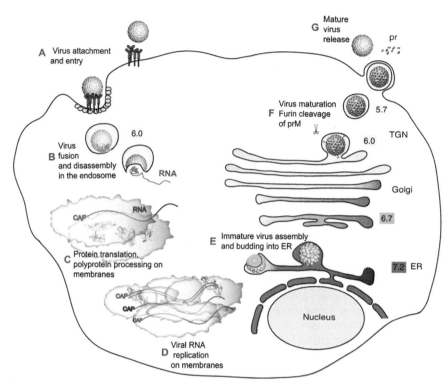

Fig. 2. Flavivirus infectious cycle, a model for ZIKV replication. A virion attaches to the surface of a susceptible and permissive host cell via interactions between the viral E protein and one or more cell-surface receptors (*A*). The virion is next internalized via clathrin-mediated endocytosis and, upon acidification of the endosome, the viral and endosomal membranes fuse, releasing the viral genome into the host cell's cytoplasm (*B*). Next, viral protein translation, RNA replication, and nascent particle assembly occur (*C*, *D*, and *E*), ultimately leading to the maturation and release of progeny particles from the cell (*F* and *G*) (*From* Perera R, Khaliq M, Kuhn RJ. Closing the door on flaviviruses: entry as a target for antiviral drug design. Antiviral Res 2008;80:11–22; with permission.)

released particles comprise a heterogeneous population of infection-competent (ie, virions) and -incompetent progeny.[26]

PATHOPHYSIOLOGY

The dynamics of ZIKV pathogenesis, the host's immune response to ZIKV infection, and the mechanisms underlying sequelae are subjects of investigation by a very large, multidisciplinary group of researchers from around the world. Our current understanding of the pathophysiology of ZIKV infection stems from a combination of in silico, in vitro, and in vivo studies, including the development of cell culture and animal models, postmortem examination of human fetal and infant remains infected with ZIKV, as well as clinical case reports that detail never-before-seen complications associated with ZIKV infection.

Infection of primary human dermal fibroblast, primary human epidermal keratinocyte, and human dendritic cell cultures demonstrate that all 3 cell types are susceptible and permissive to ZIKV infection.[28] It stands to reason that each of these cell types could participate in the amplification of ZIKV at the site of inoculation and subsequent dissemination of the virus. This study also elucidated that infection of skin fibroblast cells results in activation of innate cellular antiviral responses. By way of experimental infection of human skin biopsy specimens with ZIKV, the histopathologic features of ZIKV in skin were also assessed.[28] Studies conducted later, in 2016, demonstrated that ZIKV infects and destroys human neuronal stem cells grown as neurospheres and brain organoids, observations that helped solidify the link between fetal ZIKV infection and the development of microcephaly.[31]

Several nonhuman primate and nonprimate animal species have been evaluated to assess their suitability as models for ZIKV infection. Dudley and colleagues[32] examined the virologic and immunologic dynamics of ZIKV infection in rhesus macaques that were experimentally infected with Asian-lineage ZIKV in doses similar to those known to be delivered by the bite of infected mosquito vectors. Interestingly, the kinetics of ZIKV detection were similar to those described in human patients, with RNA being detectable in blood, urine, and other body fluids. Assessment of the immunologic response revealed the production of neutralizing antibodies, and animals appeared to be immune to reinfection following rechallenge with infectious virus 10 weeks after the initial exposure. To evaluate the effects of ZIKV infection on rhesus fetal development, 2 pregnant monkeys were included among the experimental cohorts. Conclusions of these studies have yet to be published, however. Other animal studies, including those using mice, have successfully recapitulated some pathologic features of ZIKV infection, including destruction of neuronal tissue.[33]

Postmortem analysis of ZIKV-infected human fetal and infant remains has proven pivotal in the implication of ZIKV in neuroteratogenesis. Histopathological examination of infant and placental remains from cases of lethal congenital infection has so far demonstrated that ZIKV antigens, intact viral particles, and nucleic acids are detectable in the central nervous system tissues of microcephalic fetuses and placentas. In addition, the identification of some infected cell types and affected anatomic regions (neurons and glial cells of infected infants, chorionic villi of placentas) was achieved by immunohistochemical staining for ZIKV antigens.[34]

CLINICAL PRESENTATION
Noncongenital Infections

Most ZIKV infections acquired outside of the womb are asymptomatic. Most infected individuals usually have mild symptoms, including rash, conjunctivitis, fever, and arthralgia (**Table 1**), that typically lasts 2 to 7 days. The presence of conjunctivitis differentiates ZIKV infection from that caused by DENV and CHIKV. The median duration of arthralgia among cases in Brazil was 9 days, with a range from 2 to 21 days.[35] Cases are infrequently associated with serious central nervous system syndromes such as Guillain-Barré syndrome.[36] Outside of congenitally acquired infections, fatal cases are rare, but have been reported in children and adults, and most had accompanying severe thrombocytopenia.[37,38] Before the 2015 outbreak in Latin America, ZIKV was not associated with deaths. The incubation period for ZIKV disease is not well established, but is likely to range from several days to 2 weeks.

Congenital Infections

Exposure to ZIKV during pregnancy, especially during the first trimester, is often associated with central nervous system manifestations including microcephaly, calcifications in the brain, growth restriction, and death.[39–42] The eye is also affected,

Table 1
Clinical features of Zika virus infection

Sign or Symptom	Location (Reference)				
	Yap Island[20]	Mexico[57]	Brazil[35]	Brazil[42]	Puerto Rico[37]
Fever	65[a]	96.6	36	27.8	63
Rash	90	93.3	97	100	74
Conjunctivitis	55	88.8	56	58.3	20
Arthralgia	65	Not provided	63	63.9	63
Headache	45	85.4	66	52.8	63
Myalgia	48	84.3	61	41.7	68
Retro-orbital pain	39	Not provided	45	49.3	51

[a] Percent of patients reporting.
Data from Refs.[20,35,37,42,57]

including abnormality of the retina and optic nerve.[43] Nearly a third of infected women evaluated by ultrasound showed fetal central nervous system development.[42] Fetal death was reported in 5% of cases.[42]

DIAGNOSIS
Laboratory Safety

ZIKV is classified by the US Centers for Disease Control and Prevention and the National Institutes of Health as a risk group-2 pathogen, so biosafety level-2 practices and precautions should be used for the manipulation and testing of clinical specimens as well as ZIKV cultivation.

Nucleic Acid Amplification

ZIKV RNA is usually detectable in serum by reverse-transcription-polymerase chain reaction (RT-PCR) within 2 days of symptom onset and up to 7 days after symptom onset.[44] Viral RNA is detectable in urine up to 14 days, but may appear later than it does in serum.[44,45] For this reason, testing of paired serum and urine specimens is recommended over testing a single specimen type. In a recent study of travel-associated ZIKV infections in Florida, urine was positive for ZIKV RNA in 93% of cases. Among urine specimens collected between 7 and 20 days after symptom onset, 83% were still positive by RT-PCR.[46] Among this same cohort of Zika cases with both urine and serum collected within 5 days of symptom onset, 95% of urine specimens were positive for RNA, whereas only 56% of serum specimens were positive. This study provides valuable longitudinal data on the positivity of RT-PCR from not only serum and urine but also saliva. Urine was generally positive for viral RNA through 20 days after symptom onset. RT-PCR performed on saliva had high sensitivity through 5 days after symptom onset. The sensitivity of RT-PCR performed on serum was the lowest of all 3 matrices and declined substantially by day 5 after symptom onset.[46] Testing of saliva does not extend the window of detectability, but increases the chance of detecting RNA versus blood alone.[9] ZIKV RNA is detectable in semen 2 months after symptoms and has also been detected in nasopharyngeal swabs.[47,48] Infants with suspected congenital infectious are diagnosed by RT-PCR and serologic testing. Appropriate specimens for RT-PCR testing include infant urine, cerebrospinal fluid (CSF), and serum collected within 2 days of birth.[49]

A well-designed PCR is highly specific and will not cross-react with other flaviviruses.[49] Genetic differences between ZIKV lineages can affect the sensitivity of RT-

PCR.[5,49] The diagnostic sensitivity of RT-PCR can be variable and relatively low (affected by specimen source, duration of illness, specimen collection and transport, and so forth), such that a negative PCR cannot rule out ZIKV infection. In the Yap Island outbreak, only one-third of serologically confirmed acute cases were PCR-positive by serum testing.[20] However, it should be noted that specimens in this study were collected within 10 days after onset of symptoms, well after the currently recommended window of 7 days. In a study of Zika cases imported into Europe, 3 (43%) of 7 acute phase specimens (within 5 days of illness onset) were positive by RT-PCR.[50] Finally, acute phase sera tested from 262 clinically suspected Zika cases in Brazil were tested by RT-PCR, and 119 (45.4%) were positive.[35] Cumulative data suggest that RT-PCR will be positive in about 40% to 45% of acute-phase serum samples. Unfortunately, there are no population-based studies to assess the positive and negative predictive values of RT-PCR (or serology). Most information is based on case reports, or application of laboratory methods to limited patient populations or to preselected specimen panels. To date, only a handful of commercially available ZIKV diagnostic assays have received emergency use authorization (EUA) clearance from the FDA, and those are listed in **Table 2**.

Serology

Serologic diagnosis of ZIKV infection is by detection of immunoglobulin M (IgM) antibodies in serum (or CSF in infants) using IgM antibody capture (MAC)-enzyme-linked immunosorbent assay (ELISA) with the confirmatory plaque reduction neutralization test (PRNT). IgM antibodies are usually detectable 1 week after symptom onset and remain detectable for several weeks.[46] When samples are collected at the appropriate time, MAC-ELISA is highly sensitive and can rule out infection. Because of the potential for false-negative results during the serologic window, negative IgM test results on samples collected within 2 weeks after symptom onset should be confirmed with repeat testing on a second sample collected approximately 2 to 4 weeks later. IgG has little added value over IgM; cross-reactivity with IgG response to other viruses is extensive, and IgG antibodies do not appear much sooner than IgM. PRNT is a supplemental test limited to reference public health laboratories due to technical complexity. All serologic methods, including PRNT, can cross-react with antibodies to other flaviviruses, particularly DENV. As more data are gathered on the performance of diagnostic tests for ZIKV infection, interpretation of test results may change. At one time it was thought that ZIKV and DENV virus PRNT titers at least 4-fold different could discriminate between cross-reacting antibodies.[6] However, more recent guidelines recommend that a positive PRNT titer ($\geq$10) for ZIKV together with negative PRNTs for other flaviviruses is necessary to confirm a recent ZIKV infection.[51] Commercially available ELISAs for IgG and IgM have been evaluated and those which have received EUA from the FDA are listed in **Table 2**.[52] Additional studies are needed to assess the specificity and sensitivity of these kits. In addition to serum, anti-ZIKV IgM has also been detected in amniotic fluid and CSF.[53,54]

Additional considerations for diagnostic testing are listed as follows:

- *Exposure to mosquitoes.* For asymptomatic persons, the decision on which test to perform should be based on the time between potential exposure to mosquitoes and specimen collection. For symptomatic patients, the test should be based on the time between symptom onset and specimen collection.
- *Sexual exposure.* The US Centers of Disease Control and Prevention does not recommend testing semen for the determination of risk for sexual transmission because current knowledge of the pattern of virus shedding in the male genitourinary tract is limited.[13] ZIKV can be transmitted via semen before the onset of

Table 2
Commercially available reverse-transcription-polymerase chain reaction and serological test kits that have been granted emergency use authorization by the US Food and Drug Administration (as of September 21, 2016)

Test Device Name	Test Method	Manufacturer	Notes
Molecular methods			
Abbot RealTime ZIKA Assay	rRT-PCR	Abbott Molecular, Inc	For qualitative detection of ZIKV RNA
Aptima Zika Virus Assay	TMA	Hologic, Inc	For qualitative detection of ZIKV RNA
Lightmix Zika rRT-PCR Test	rRT-PCR	Roche Molecular Systems, Inc	For qualitative detection of ZIKV RNA
RealStar Zika Virus RT-PCR Kit	rRT-PCR	Altona Diagnostics GmbH	For qualitative detection of ZIKV RNA
Trioplex Real-time RT-PCR Assay	rRT-PCR	CDC	For qualitative detection of CHIKV, DENV, and ZIKV RNA. Not available for commercial distribution
VERSANT Zika RNA 1.0 Assay (kPCR) Kit	rRT-PCR	Siemens Healthcare Diagnostics, Inc.	For qualitative detection of ZIKV RNA
xMAP MultiFLEX Zika RNA Assay	RT-PCR/BH	Luminex Corporation	For qualitative detection of ZIKV RNA
Serologic methods			
Zika MAC-ELISA	ELISA	CDC	For qualitative detection of ZIKV IgM antibodies in serum
ZIKV Detect IgM Capture ELISA	ELISA	InBios International, Inc.	For qualitative detection of ZIKV IgM antibodies in serum

Abbreviations: BH, bead hybridization; rRT-PCR, real-time reverse-transcription polymerase chain reaction; TMA, transcription-mediated amplification.

Data from Food and Drug Administration. Emergency use authorization–Zika virus EUA information. Available at: http://www.fda.gov/EmergencyPreparedness/Counterterrorism/MedicalCountermeasures/MCMLegalRegulatoryandPolicyFramework/ucm182568.htm. Accessed September 21, 2016.

symptoms as well as long after symptoms resolve.[22] The type of testing performed on a potentially exposed person should be dictated by the time between exposure or symptoms and when the specimen was collected.

- *In utero/newborn infants.* RT-PCR testing of placenta, CSF, urine, and serum from the infant is recommended. Detection of ZIKV RNA in the placenta alone cannot distinguish between maternal and congenital infection. Brain tissue is recommended postmortem. ZIKV RNA is detectable in these specimens for weeks to months following initial infection.[53,55] In addition, IgM is usually detectable in CSF of microcephalic infants at birth.[54]

Cultivation

A number of cell lines, including primary nonhuman primate kidney cells and established cell lines such as Vero and A549 cells, are susceptible and permissive to infection with ZIKV. Generally, cells exhibit cytopathic effect (rounding of cells and degeneration of the cell monolayer) within 1 week of infection. Isolates can be identified by various molecular methods, including PCR and nucleotide sequencing. Although useful for epidemiological and basic research purposes, cultivation is not practical for routine diagnosis, as a majority of clinical laboratories no longer perform viral culture, and most of those that do cannot reliably identify ZIKV from cultured cells.

Differential Diagnosis

Patients with ZIKV infection typically present with a systemic febrile rash illness that may share some additional features with dengue and chikungunya fevers, including arthralgia, myalgias, and headache. The geographic distribution of these viruses overlaps with that of ZIKV. The differential diagnosis also includes infections caused by influenza virus, *Plasmodium* spp, *Leptospira* spp, WNV, and YFV. The differential diagnosis of fetal growth restriction and central nervous system manifestations includes human cytomegalovirus infection, toxoplasmosis, syphilis, and rubella.

TREATMENT AND PREVENTION

There are no clinically approved antiviral agents for treatment of ZIKV infections. There is currently no vaccine approved by the FDA. Approaches for vaccine development based on those used for other flaviviruses have been discussed.[56] Prevention of ZIKV virus infection is accomplished by avoiding mosquito bites. ZIKV is transmitted by *Aedes* spp mosquitoes, which feed during the day. Avoidance measures include wearing clothing to cover skin, application of insect repellent, staying indoors with adequate physical barriers (windows, screens), sleeping under a mosquito bed net, as well as additional measures outlined in guidance documents.[13] Sexual transmission of ZIKV can be prevented by the use of condoms during sex, or abstinence from sex. Measures to reduce the risk of transfusion-transmitted ZIKV infection include self-deferral and screening of blood donors. There are currently no FDA-approved ZIKV nucleic acid amplification tests for screening of blood donations; however, the FDA stipulates that blood collection centers can use investigational individual donor nucleic acid tests. An investigational test is being used under an investigational new drug application to screen blood donations in regions with active mosquito-borne transmission.[57]

SUMMARY

Although ZIKV shares some features with other flaviviruses, the ability to spread via sexual intercourse and its ability to cause birth defects is, so far, unique. Although most ZIKV infections are asymptomatic and most symptomatic infections resolve without complications, the association of ZIKV infection with fetal neurologic defects is alarming and is driving much of the demand for diagnostic testing and patient screening. Much remains to be understood about the pathogenesis and epidemiology of ZIKV as well as the laboratory diagnosis of ZIKV infection. Guidance on the use and interpretation of laboratory tests, and the clinical management of infected patients, continues to evolve as more information becomes available, which currently occurs on a nearly daily basis.

REFERENCES

1. Campos GS, Bandeira AC, Sardi SI. Zika virus outbreak, Bahia, Brazil (letter). Emerg Infect Dis 2015;21(10):1885–6.
2. Hennessey M, Fischer M, Staples JE. Zika virus spreads to new areas—region of the Americas, May 2015-January 2016. MMWR Morb Mortal Wkly Rep 2016;65: 55–8.

3. Dick GW, Kitchen SF, Haddow AJ. Zika virus. I. isolations and serological specificity. Trans R Soc Trop Med Hyg 1952;46(5):509–20.
4. MacNamara FN. Zika virus: a report on three cases of human infection during an epidemic of jaundice in Nigeria. Trans R Soc Trop Med Hyg 1954;48(2):139–45.
5. Waggoner JJ, Pinsky BA. Zika virus: diagnostics for an emerging pandemic threat. J Clin Microbiol 2016;54(4):860–7.
6. Lanciotti RS, Kosoy OL, Laven JJ, et al. Genetic and serologic properties of Zika virus associated with an epidemic, Yap State, Micronesia, 2007. Emerg Infect Dis 2008;14(8):1232–9.
7. Cao-Lormeau V-M, Roche C, Teissier A, et al. Zika virus, French Polynesia, South Pacific, 2013. Emerg Infect Dis 2014;20(6):1085–6.
8. Atif M, Azeem M, Sarwar MR, et al. Zika virus disease: a current review of the literature. Infection 2016;44(6):695–705.
9. Musso D, Roche C, Nhan TX, et al. Detection of Zika virus in saliva. J Clin Virol 2015;68:53–5.
10. World Health Organization. Pacific syndromic surveillance report. Week 13, ending 30th March, 2014. Manila (Philippines): World Health Organization Western Pacific Region; 2014.
11. European Centre for Disease Prevention and Control. Monitoring current threats: ECDC communicable disease threats report (CTDR), week 11/2014. Stockholm (Sweden): European Centre for Disease Prevention and Control; 2014.
12. Lednicky J, Beau De Rochars VM, El Badry M, et al. Zika virus outbreak in Haiti in 2014: molecular and clinical data. PLoS Negl Trop Dis 2016;10(4):e0004687.
13. Centers for Disease Control and Prevention. Zika virus. Available at: http://www.cdc.gov/zika/index.html. Accessed September 21, 2016.
14. Haddow AD, Schuh AJ, Yasuda CY, et al. Genetic characterization of Zika virus strains: geographic expansion of the Asian lineage. PLoS Negl Trop Dis 2012;6(2):e1477.
15. Darwish MA, Hoogstraal H, Roberts TJ, et al. A sero-epidemiological survey for certain arboviruses (Togaviridae) in Pakistan. Trans R Soc Trop Med Hyg 1983;77:442–5.
16. Olson JG, Ksiazek TG, Gubler DJ, et al. A survey for arboviral antibodies in sera of humans and animals in Lombok, Republic of Indonesia. Ann Trop Med Parasitol 1983;77(2):131–7.
17. Vorou R. Zika virus, vectors, reservoirs, amplifying hosts, and their potential to spread worldwide: what we know and what we should investigate urgently. Int J Infect Dis 2016;48:85–90.
18. Kading RC, Schountz T. Flavivirus infections in bats: potential role in Zika virus ecology. Am J Trop Med Hyg 2016;95(5):993–6.
19. Guerbois M, Fernandez-Salas I, Azar SR, et al. Outbreak of Zika virus infection, Chiapas State, Mexico, 2015, and first confirmed transmission by Aedes aegypti in the Americas. J Infect Dis 2016;214(9):1349–56.
20. Duffy MR, Chen T-H, Hancock WT, et al. Zika virus outbreak on Yap Island, Federated States of Micronesia. N Engl J Med 2009;360:2536–43.
21. Grard G, Caron M, Mombo IM, et al. Zika virus in Gabon (Central Africa)—2007: a new threat from Aedes albopictus? PLoS Negl Trop Dis 2014;8(2):e2681.
22. Foy BD, Kobylinski KC, Chilson-Foy JL, et al. Probable non-vector-borne transmission of Zika virus, Colorado, USA. Emerg Infect Dis 2011;17(5):880–2.
23. Davidson A, Slavinski S, Komoto K, et al. Suspected female-to-male sexual transmission of Zika virus—New York City, 2016. MMWR Morb Mortal Wkly Rep 2016;65(28):716–7.

24. Agência Saúde. MICROCEFALIA Ministério da Saúde divulga boletim epidemiologico. 2015. Available at: http://portalsaude.saude.gov.br/index.php/cidadao/principal/agencia-saude/20805-ministerio-da-saude-divulga-boletim-epidemiologico. Accessed September 21, 2016.

25. Barjas-Castro ML, Angerami RN, Cunha MS, et al. Probable transfusion-transmitted Zika virus in Brazil. Transfusion 2016;56(7):1684–8.

26. Sirohi D, Chen Z, Sun L, et al. The 3.8 Å resolution cryo-EM structure of Zika virus. Science 2016;352(6284):467–70.

27. Perera-Lecoin M, Meertens L, Carnec X, et al. 2013 Flavivirus entry receptors: an update. Viruses 2013;6(1):69–88.

28. Hamel R, Dejarnac O, Wichit S, et al. Biology of Zika virus infection in human skin cells. J Virol 2015;89:8880–96.

29. Buckley A, Gould EA. Detection of virus-specific antigen in the nuclei or nucleoli of cells infected with Zika or Langat virus. J Gen Virol 1988;69(Pt 8):1913–20.

30. Kuhn RJ, Dowd KA, Post CB, et al. Shake, rattle, and roll: impact of the dynamics of flavivirus particles on their interactions with the host. Virology 2015;479-480:508–17.

31. Garcez PP, Loiola EC, Madeiro da Costa R, et al. Zika virus impairs growth in human neurospheres and brain organoids. Science 2016;352(6287):816–8.

32. Dudley DM, Aliota MT, Mohr EL, et al. A rhesus macaque model of Asian-lineage Zika virus infection. Nat Commun 2016;7:12204.

33. Li H, Saucedo-Cuevas L, Reglas-Nava JA, et al. Zika virus infects neural progenitors in the adult mouse brain and alters proliferation. Cell Stem Cell 2016;19(5):593–8.

34. Martines RB, Bhatnagar J, de Oliveira Ramos AM, et al. Pathology of congenital Zika syndrome in Brazil: a case series. Lancet 2016;388(10047):898–904.

35. Brasil P, Calvet GA, Siqueira AM, et al. 2016 Zika virus outbreak in Rio de Janeiro, Brazil: clinical characterization, epidemiological and virological aspects. PLoS Negl Trop Dis 2016;10(4):e0004636.

36. Brasil P, Sequeira PC, Freitas AD, et al. Guillain-Barré syndrome associated with Zika virus infection. Lancet 2016;387(10026):1482.

37. Dirlikov E, Ryff KR, Torres-Aponte J, et al. Update: ongoing Zika virus transmission—Puerto Rico, November 1, 2015–April 14, 2016. MMWR Morb Mortal Wkly Rep 2016;65(17):451–5.

38. Sarmiento-Ospina A, Vásquez-Serna H, Jimenez-Canizales CE, et al. Zika virus associated deaths in Colombia. Lancet Infect Dis 2016;16(5):523–4.

39. Noronha LD, Zanluca C, Azevedo ML, et al. Zika virus damages the human placental barrier and presents marked fetal neurotropism. Mem Inst Oswaldo Cruz 2016;111(5):287–93.

40. de Fatima Vasco Aragao M, van der Linden V, Brainer-Lima AM, et al. Clinical features of neuroimaging (CT and MRI) findings in presumed Zika virus related congenital infection and microcephaly: retrospective case series study. BMJ 2016;353:i1901.

41. Microcephaly Epidemic Research Group1. Microcephaly in infants, Pernambuco State, Brazil, 2015. Emerg Infect Dis 2016;22(6):1090–3.

42. Brasil P, Pereira JP Jr, Raja Gabaglia C, et al. Zika virus infection in pregnant women in Rio je Janeiro—preliminary report. N Engl J Med 2016;375(24):2321–34.

43. Miranda HA 2nd, Costa MC, Frazão MA, et al. Expanded spectrum of congenital ocular findings in microcephaly with presumed Zika infection. Ophthalmology 2016;123(8):1788–94.

44. Campos Rde M, Cirne-Santos C, Meira GL, et al. Prolonged detection of Zika virus RNA in urine samples during the ongoing Zika virus epidemic in Brazil. J Clin Virol 2016;77:69–70.
45. Gourinat AC, O'Connor O, Calvez E, et al. Detection of Zika virus in urine. Emerg Infect Dis 2015;21(1):84–6.
46. Bingham AM, Cone M, Mock V, et al. Comparison of test results for Zika virus RNA in urine, serum, and saliva specimens from persons with travel-associated Zika virus disease—Florida, 2016. MMWR Morb Mortal Wkly Rep 2016;65(18):475–8.
47. Atkinson B, Hearn P, Afrough B, et al. Detection of Zika virus in semen. Emerg Infect Dis 2016;22(5):940.
48. Fonseca K, Meatherall B, Zarra D, et al. First case of Zika virus infection in a returning Canadian traveler. Am J Trop Med Hyg 2014;91(4):1035–8.
49. Russell K, Oliver SE, Lewis L, et al. Update: interim guidance for the evaluation and management of infants with possible congenital Zika virus infection—United States, August 2016. MMWR Morb Mortal Wkly Rep 2016;65(11):286–9.
50. De Smet B, Van den Bossche D, van de Werve C, et al. Confirmed Zika virus infection in a Belgian traveler returning from Guatemala, and the diagnostic challenges of imported cases into Europe. J Clin Virol 2016;80:8–11.
51. Rabe IB, Staples JE, Villanueva J, et al. Interim guidance for interpretation of Zika virus antibody test results. MMWR Morb Mortal Wkly Rep 2016;65(21):543–6.
52. Huzly D, Hanselmann I, Schmidt-Chanasit J, et al. High specificity of a novel Zika virus ELISA in European patients after exposure to different flaviviruses. Euro Surveill 2016;21(16).
53. Calvet G, Aguiar RS, Melo AS, et al. Detection and sequencing of Zika virus from amniotic fluid of fetuses with microcephaly in Brazil: a case study. Lancet Infect Dis 2016;16(6):653–60.
54. Cordeiro MT, Pena LJ, Brito CA, et al. Positive IgM for Zika virus in the cerebrospinal fluid of 30 neonates with microcephaly in Brazil. Lancet 2016;387(10030):1811–2.
55. Mlakar J, Korva M, Tul N, et al. Zika virus associated with microcephaly. N Engl J Med 2016;374(10):951–8.
56. Weaver SC, Costa F, Garcia-Blanco MA, et al. Zika virus: history, emergence, biology, and prospects for control. Antiviral Res 2016;130:69–80.
57. Jimenez Corona ME, De la Garza Barroso AL, Rodriguez Martinez JC, et al. Clinical and epidemiological characterization of laboratory-confirmed autochthonous cases of Zika virus disease in Mexico. PLoS Curr 2016;8.

Ebola Virus Disease

An Update on Epidemiology, Symptoms, Laboratory Findings, Diagnostic Issues, and Infection Prevention and Control Issues for Laboratory Professionals

Colin S. Brown, FRCPath[a,b,]*, Stephen Mepham, FRCPath[c], Robert J. Shorten, PhD[d,e]

KEYWORDS

- Ebola • Viral hemorrhagic fever • Safety • Preparedness

KEY POINTS

- The 2013-2016 Ebola virus disease (EVD) outbreak in West Africa was unprecedented in both scale and location.
- The large number of patients infected has led to an increased knowledge base about EVD, though much remains to be elucidated.
- The experience in the countries directly affected, as well as those in resource-rich settings which cared for imported cases, has highlighted the requirement for clear diagnostic, management, and infection prevention and control pathways in dealing with such infections.
- Facilities should be aware of blood abnormalities, clinical manifestations, and epidemiological risks for EVD acquisition, and national recommendations regarding processing of potentially-infected clinical samples.

Funding Support & Conflict of Interest: No funding. The authors have nothing to disclose.
[a] Weston Education Centre, King's Sierra Leone Partnership, King's Centre for Global Health, King's Health Partners, King's College London, London SE5 9RJ, UK; [b] National Infection Service, Public Health England, London, UK; [c] Department of Infection, Royal Free London NHS Foundation Trust, London, UK; [d] Public Health Laboratory Manchester, Manchester Royal Infirmary, Manchester, UK; [e] Department of Infection, Centre for Clinical Microbiology, University College London, London, UK
* Corresponding author. Weston Education Centre, King's Sierra Leone Partnership, King's Centre for Global Health, King's Health Partners, King's College London, London SE5 9RJ, UK.
E-mail address: colinbrown@doctors.net.uk

HISTORY OF EBOLA VIRUS DISEASE

Ebola virus disease (EVD) has historically been one of the world's most feared diseases. First discovered with simultaneous outbreaks in Nzara, South Sudan, and Yambuka, Democratic Republic of the Congo (previously called Zaire), by 2013 there had been more than 1700 cases with a case fatality rate ranging from 25% to 90%.[1] There are 4 strains of virus that affect humans, with Zaire ebolavirus the most commonly seen in outbreaks (the others being Sudan, Bundigbugyo, Taï Forest). Reston ebolavirus causes infection in nonhuman primates and swine, although there is serologic evidence of response to subclinical infection in humans.[2]

Until 2014, EVD was thought to be a disease that was too rapidly fatal to lead to widespread outbreaks. It was thought to be a localized, rural disease in Central Africa, with limited risk of transfer to large urban centers, with subsequent risk on onward regional or global dispersal. The largest outbreak seen to date was in Gulu, Uganda, in 2000, with 425 cases with a case fatality rate of 53%.[1] The 2013 to 2016 EVD Outbreak in West Africa radically challenged those assumptions. Recognized in early March 2014 in Guinea and Liberia and in May 2014 in Sierra Leone, with an index case thought to have arisen in Guinea in December 2013, by the time the World Health Organization (WHO) declared the conclusion of the Public Health Emergency of International Concern in March 2016,[3] more than 28,000 people had been infected, with more than 11,00 deaths.[4] Cases were imported into, some with localized onward transmission in Mali (8), Nigeria (20), the United States (2), the United Kingdom (1), Senegal (1), and Spain (1),[4] along with the repatriation of a further 24 patients to the United States and Europe.[5] Early modeling in September 2014 suggested that many countries could expect imported cases based on existing air traffic routes, with West African and European countries being most at risk (with up to 50% likelihood suggested for Ghana).[6] With a reduction in service as airlines canceled travel, by the end of 2014, this was revised to a risk of approximately 3 travelers infected with Ebola virus (EBOV) departing the 3 most affected countries via commercial flights each month.[7] Many countries implemented returning traveler surveillance schemes. Models suggested that these may detect some and identify the remainder through dedicated information and passenger follow-up.[8] Although the projected number of imported cases were not seen, facilities worldwide were needed to make adequate preparations for advance management of cases, including appropriate isolation, testing, and treatment of suspected patients with viral hemorrhagic fevers (VHF).[9]

In this review, the authors highlight the epidemiology, symptoms, laboratory findings, diagnostics, and infection prevention and control issues that will be useful for laboratory professionals managing such suspect cases.

RISK ASSESSMENT OF THE RETURNING TRAVELER

Within the United Kingdom, the Advisory Committee on Dangerous Pathogens (ACDP), an expert committee of the Department of Health, produces guidelines for the recommended assessment and management of returning febrile travelers at risk of Hazard Group 4 pathogens (VHF and similar human infectious diseases of high consequence, also known as high containment pathogens). These guidelines have been recently updated to allow for more local processing of samples with recognition that the vast majority of patients who trigger a VHF screen will have an alternative diagnosis.[10] The ACDP guidelines have clear algorithms on which questions should be asked in order to ascertain whether VHFs should be considered within a differential diagnosis; these include initial screening questions on the presence or history of a fever greater than 37.5°C, and development of symptoms within 21 days of leaving a

VHF endemic country (the incubation period of EVD is 2–21 days). If the answer to these is negative, VHF can be excluded as a possibility. If the answer is positive, risk stratification is determined on subsequent questions, including whether the individual has had recent contact with bodily fluids or clinical specimens from a patient or laboratory animal known or strongly suspected to have VHF; has traveled to an area known to have a current VHF outbreak; has lived or worked in basic rural conditions in an area where Lassa Fever is endemic; has visited caves or mines, or had contact with or eaten primates, antelopes or bats, in a Marburg/Ebola endemic area; or has traveled to a Crimean-Congo hemorrhagic fever (CCHF) endemic area where it is endemic and sustained a tick bite or crushed a tick with their bare hands or had close involvement with animal slaughter. If an obvious alternative diagnosis has been made such as tick typhus, then they can be managed accordingly, although those with confirmed malaria should be considered at risk of VHF coinfection.[10]

The use of advisory services for centers unfamiliar with such risk assessment is recommended, such as the Imported Fever Service within the United Kingdom, an around-the-clock clinical advisory and specialist diagnostic service for medical professionals managing febrile travelers, which provides access to a 24-hour on-call molecular diagnostic service for VHF.[11] In the United States, the Centers for Disease Control and Prevention (CDC) produced specific guidance for suspected EVD-infected cases during the West African outbreak, although this was retired following its cessation.[12] There are general EVD recommendations that highlight epidemiologic exposure as key in determining the risk of evaluating patients.[13] European countries such as Germany also have robust guidelines that cover the risk assessment of returning travelers suspected with having EVD, that as well as clinical aspects of diagnosis and management include infection control measures such as disinfection, disposal of waste, and management of waste water.[14] The German definitions are broadly similar to the United Kingdom for EVD risk assessment with regards to potential exposure, although they recommend using a temperature of greater than 38.5°C.

Readers are encouraged to familiarize themselves with their national guidelines and adapt them for local practice, including strict attention to patient management once presenting to local health center. Within the United Kingdom, this has involved creating patient flow pathways within each hospital regarding the exact areas they are received and managed on presentation to emergency department, which rooms they will be processed in, suitable areas for donning and doffing personal protective equipment, the collection of blood samples, transport to pathology departments, assessments of which routine tests can be processed locally, and disposal of body fluids and waste. Guidance was produced by the College of Emergency Medicine and Public Health England[15]; the CDC has produced similar facility preparedness guidelines.[16]

SPECTRUM OF CLINICAL DISEASE PRESENTATION

Given the large number of patients who have been diagnosed with EVD over the past 3 years, there is increasing evidence regarding the spectrum of clinical disease and prominent laboratory features. Unlike CCHF,[17] the most geographically widespread and prevalent VHF, EVD usually causes severe illness in those infected. Disease presentation begins with nonspecific symptoms, such as fever, severe fatigue and weakness, and headache, sometime accompanied with a maculopapular rash; progresses to a gastrointestinal phase with nausea, vomiting, diarrhea, abdominal pain, hiccups; and in some cases progresses with shock, delirium, secondary infections, and rarely, severe bleeding as late complications.[18,19] The undifferentiated early illness therefore makes separation from other infectious etiology very difficult. Furthermore, fever was not reported in large numbers of patients: 17% in one large case series from Sierra Leone[20] and 13% in another,[21] and only 36% had documented fever in a smaller study.[22] Attempts at defining combinations of symptoms to increase discriminatory power have proven difficult, with slightly different findings. One setting found that 3 or more symptoms of intense fatigue, confusion, conjunctivitis, hiccups, diarrhea, or vomiting 3-fold increased the likelihood of confirmed EVD, although the sensitivity was low.[20] Another found that the greater the number of either having an ill contact, diarrhea, anorexia, myalgia, dysphagia, or absence of abdominal pain, was predictive of disease.[23] A further group found simply the more symptoms patients presented with (at least 6 out of 21), the greater the likelihood of EVD,[24] highlighting the difficulty in prediction based on symptoms alone. In children, clinical features are notably more challenging and the suspected EVD WHO case definition is broader than for adults.[25] Again, lack of fever is common: one study highlighted 25% of children were afebrile on admission.[26]

Facilities should also be aware of the clinical sequelae of EVD syndrome, which include arthralgia, ocular symptoms including uveitis, fatigue, abdominal pain, headache, auditory symptoms and sleep disturbance, alopecia, skin disorders, anemia, and back pain.[27–29] Prior outbreaks with case-control studies have also reported myalgia and anorexia as common early sequelae.[30] Meningoencephalitis with recrudescence in cerebrospinal fluid[31] and in blood,[32] and ocular involvement including reactivation of virus in the eye,[33] have been reported. There is also a case report of asymptomatic viral shedding in pregnancy,[34] and a recent meta-analysis estimated asymptomatic household seroconversion at 27%.[35] Viable seminal carriage in survivors has previously been reported up to 82 days after infection, with viral RNA detected 284 days after infection.[36] A recent article suggested that EBOV was detected in seminal fluid 531 days after symptoms developed, with good evidence that the virus was viable caused sexual transmission about 470 days after disease onset.[37] EBOV has been cultured from urine and breast milk 26 and 15 days after illness onset, and viral RNA has been detected in urine, aqueous humor, sweat, semen, breast milk, feces, and conjunctival fluid, as well as in vaginal secretions from 15 to 272 days,[38] although one recent study showed multiple body sites tested negative for RNA after a median of 140 days.[39] Sexual contact with survivors has been reported as the mode of transmission in several cases in West Africa following declarations that countries were EVD free.[36]

Together this emphasizes the importance of epidemiologic considerations and detailed medical and travel history taking in assessing febrile patients: reassuringly there has never been a reported case of reactivation in a person not known to have had previous EVD.

ABNORMAL LABORATORY FINDINGS AND PROGNOSTIC FACTORS

There are several abnormal blood parameters, although not pathognomonic of VHF or EVD, which may influence further risk assessment if patients were not already risk assessed in advance of routine laboratory diagnostic processing and subsequently were found to have traveled to an at-risk area. In cases treated in a resource-rich setting, prominent laboratory findings were hypoalbuminemia, hyponatremia, hypokalemia, hypocalcemia, and hypomagnesemia, alongside transaminitis, thrombocytopenia, lymphopenia, and elevated lactate and creatine kinase levels.[5] In African settings, kidney and liver insults, alongside raised hematocrit, thrombocytopenia, leukopenia, granulocytosis, increased bleeding time, hypoglycemia, abnormal serum potassium, and raised C-reactive protein have been reported.[40,41] One key difficulty is distinguishing these abnormal blood parameters from those associated with other febrile illnesses, such as malaria, leptospirosis, Dengue fever, or severe bacterial sepsis such as staphylococcal septicemia.

Several large case series have identified prognostic markers of severe disease. A recent meta-analysis of these highlighted that symptoms that predicted mortality included hemorrhage, abdominal pain, vomiting, diarrhea, cough, sore throat, and conjunctivitis.[42] Coma, confusion, chest pain, hiccups, and respiratory distress have also been associated with worse outcomes as has age, and lesser duration of symptom onset to presentation.[43–45] In children, signs significantly associated with mortality were fever, vomiting, and diarrhea. Hiccups, bleeding, and confusion were exclusively observed in children who died in one study setting.[26] Nucleic acid amplification tests (NAATs) provide not only a qualitative positive/negative result but also an indication of the number of virions within the sample. High viremia is a common prognostic factor of mortality in both adults and children,[26,40,46–48] along with severe kidney injury and hepatitis.[40] These predictors of fatal outcomes are very similar to other VHFs, such as severe cases of CCHF; a recent review of CCHF highlighted somnolence, bleeding, thrombocytopenia, elevated liver enzymes, and prolonged bleeding times as the most common predictors of poor clinical outcomes, along with viremia.[49] Mortality varies by treatment setting: 18.5% in a resource-rich setting,[5] and between 40% and 90% in West Africa.[18]

EBOLA VIRUS DISEASE DIAGNOSTICS

The preferred diagnostic method is the detection of viral RNA using NAATs. Molecular assays have advantages over the previous technologies of enzyme immunoassay, electron microscopy, and immunofluorescence, including increased sensitivity, specificity, and faster turnaround. Several of these molecular assays are available commercially or as in-house assays performed by specialized reference centers (**Table 1**). Because of the hazardous nature of the viruses involved and the level of manual manipulation required, nucleic acid extraction is usually performed inside a containment laboratory before amplification and detection. This process allows additional differential diagnoses to be investigated at the same time. In the United Kingdom, travelers returning from VHF-endemic areas will be tested for a panel of likely pathogens according to the Imported Fever Service discussions.[11] Assays for other geographically relevant diseases, which may present in a similar fashion (such as malaria, Lassa fever, or dengue), are performed in parallel. The Public Health England (PHE) Rare and Imported Pathogens Laboratory (RIPL) perform a range of these molecular assays according to patient epidemiology, including pan-Ebola[1] and Ebola Zaire specific[2] NAATs. Results are obtained as rapidly as possible to permit the deescalation of patient isolation and specimen containment or, if positive, expedite transfer to specialized centers.

Serial viral load testing may be useful in monitoring disease progression. NAAT testing of other anatomic sites in the convalescent phase may inform the infection prevention and control risk assessment before patient deisolation, as evidenced by culture and polymerase chain reaction (PCR) above; more data are needed to understand the relationship between positive tests for EBOV RNA in these sites and risk of disease transmission.

Before the West Africa EVD outbreak, all UK testing for EVD and other imported differential diagnoses were performed at RIPL. There was a need to increase testing capacity and reduce turnaround times due to the size of the West Africa outbreak, and therefore, the large number of individuals entering the United Kingdom who were

Table 1
Summary of diagnostic nucleic acid amplification tests for Ebola virus disease

Company & Assay Name	Assay Target[a]	Limit of Viral Detection	Maximum Time to Obtaining Result	Stage of Development/Reference
Altona (Hamburg, Germany): 2 Assays				
a. Real Star Filovirus Screen	Real-time NAAT targeting the L gene of all 5 Ebola viruses	3.16 copies/μL[b]	4 h	CE-IVD marked
b. Real Star Ebolavirus	Real-time NAAT for detection and differentiation of all 5 Ebola viruses	116–675 copies/μL[b] (1250 copies/mL)	4 h	Emergency use authorization from FDA[50]
Biocartis (Mechelen, Belgium), Janssen Diagnostics (Raritan, NJ, USA), & the Institute for Tropical Medicine in Antwerp (Belgium), Idylla system	Real-time NAAT on a fully automated molecular diagnostic platform using 0.2 mL of blood	465 PFU/mL[b]	100 min	CE-IVD marked in Europe
BioMerieux (Marcy-l'Étoile, France), BioFire Film Array Biothreat-E test	Real-time NAAT for detection of ZEBOV blood and urine within approximately 1 h	600,000 PFU/mL[b] 400 TCID$_{50}$/mL	2 h	Emergency use authorization from FDA[51,52]
Cepheid (Sunnyvale, CA, USA), Xpert Ebola	Real-time NAAT for detection of ZEBOV blood and urine	232 copies/mL[b]	100 min	Emergency use authorization from FDA[53]
Non commercial	Cell phone sized, one-stage RT-PCR for ZEBOV, including melt-curve analysis (targets not reported)	Not quantified	<1 h, excluding nucleic extraction	[54]
LA-200 (turbidimeter): Eiken Chemical Co Ltd, Tokyo, Japan & Genie III (fluorescence detection): OptiGene, West Sussex, UK	RT-LAMP with multiple targets in the trailer and NP regions of ZEBOV	Approx. 600 copies per assay	35 min, excluding nucleic acid extraction	[55]

Panning assay	Noncommercial pan-Filovirus multiplex NAAT targeting L gene	10 copies per assay	4 h	[56]
Platinum nanoparticles incorporated volumetric bar-chart chip (PtNPs-V-Chip)	Noncommercial; colorimetric detection of nucleic acid using monoclonal antibodies, hybridization chain reaction, and platinum nanoparticles	Not quantified	Not stated	[57]
Roche (Basel, Switzerland) & TIB MOLBIOL GmbH (Berlin, Germany), LightMix Ebola Zaire Rt-PCR	Real-time PCR targeting the L gene. Up to 96 results in just over 3 h and is compatible with LightCycler 480 or Cobas z 480 instruments	4781 PFU/mL[b] 1250 copies/mL	>3 h	Emergency use authorization from FDA. CE marked, but has not yet been cleared or approved for general use by the FDA[50]
Thermos Thermal Cycler	RT-PCR targeting GP, NP, & VP24 genes performed using Thermos flasks and detection using gel electrophoresis	Not quantified	<1 h, excluding nucleic extraction	[58]
Trombley assay	Noncommercial pan-VHF multiplex NAAT	0.001–1.0 PFU/PCR	4 h	[59]

Abbreviations: CE, Conformité Européene; FDA, US Food and Drug Administration; GP, glycoprotein; IVD, in vitro diagnostic medical devices; NP, nucleoprotein; PFU, plaque forming unit; RT, reverse transcription; $TCID_{50}$/mL, 50% tissue culture infections dose; ZEBOV, Zaire Ebola virus.
[a] If available in published literature or from the manufacturer.
[b] Manufacturer's data.

assessed to be at risk of EVD. PHE introduced diagnostic testing to several regional centers with the use of a commercial assay (Biofire Film Array; BioMérieux, Marcy l'Etoile, France). Samples therefore had to be safely transported to the closest designated laboratory using packaging UN2814 (category A) or UN3373 (category B) depending on the risk assessment via a preapproved courier service.[10] Laboratories will need to have detailed algorithms in place for transport of suspected samples to regional referral testing centers.

PATHOGEN HANDLING

EBOV is categorized as a high-hazard pathogen that is handled at Biosafety Level 4 (BSL-4) in the United States[60] and is designated as a Hazard Group 4 Pathogen in the United Kingdom.[10] As such, appropriate laboratory facilities are required to examine samples that may contain these viruses. These laboratory suites must be highly secure with restricted access. Air-handling is carefully managed using pressure gradients and air filtration to ensure the containment of these pathogens, with meticulous control and inactivation of hazardous waste. Staff are highly trained to be able to work at this level of containment. Individuals who manipulate these samples are protected from infection with these viruses in 1 of 2 ways: either by the isolation of the scientist, via suited systems, or by isolating the specimens themselves with microbiological safety cabinets. Containment facilities such as these are expensive and labor intensive to build, commission, maintain, and resource, so work on such high hazard pathogens are usually restricted to a few national or regional centers in resource-rich settings. In the United Kingdom, bespoke hazard group 3 + pathogen laboratories are also located within the High Level Isolation Units (HLIU), Royal Free Hospital (London), and the Royal Victoria Infirmary (Newcastle), the national centers for managing confirmed cases of VHF. These units do not provide Containment Level 4 facilities, but they enable staff to provide pathology assays to exclude alternative diagnoses, such as rapid malaria diagnostics and blood cultures, and to support patient clinical management decisions. These facilities are staffed by trained scientific staff and are available at all times. The United States has many sites that are accredited as Ebola Treatment Centers, which require that "laboratory procedures/protocols, dedicated space, if possible, possible point-of-care testing, equipment, staffing, reagents, training, and specimen transport are in place."[61] Germany has several regional centers with BSL-4 capacity, and all diagnostics are recommended to be performed in such laboratories following shipping according to UN2814.[14]

LOCAL MANAGEMENT BEFORE CONFIRMATION OF VIRAL HEMORRHAGIC FEVER

Although diagnostic assays are awaited from reference facilities, it is important to manage the patient appropriately. Performing pathology assays that measure the complications of EVD is imperative to monitor disease progression and assist clinical teams to correct such abnormalities. Although diagnostic assays are awaited, differing country guidelines recommend what tests can be performed locally. In the United Kingdom, the ACDP states that although EVD diagnostic assays are awaited, supportive pathology assays may be analyzed safely at Containment Level 2 using routine processes and autoanalyzers following appropriate risk assessment.[10] Indeed, requesting clinicians need only inform the testing laboratory should the patient be categorized as "high possibility of VHF." Laboratories may then make provision to safely store the samples until a diagnosis is made as laboratory waste containing a VHF should be classified as Category A and should be discarded appropriately following analysis.[62] To ensure a safe system of work, protocols for machine decontamination, maintenance, management of spillages, and waste disposal must be in place and followed, taking into consideration manufacturers' recommendations. Autoanalyzers should be disinfected following local procedures after sample processing and before scheduled maintenance.[10] In addition to the handling of clinical waste, some slight variations to routine laboratory processing are recommended when processing samples from a patient categorized as "high possibility of VHF." Blood film slides for malaria should be prepared in a microbiological safety cabinet or alternatively facial protection should be used: this is to provide protection from potential splashes. The use of point of care (POC) analyzers, in particular blood gas analyzers, is not recommended.[10] Before any facility processing specimens for patients with suspected EVD, the CDC recommended that laboratory managers and safety officers must perform a site-specific risk assessment to "determine the potential for exposure from sprays, splashes, or aerosols generated during all laboratory processes, procedures, and activities."[63] German guidelines allow for EVD diagnostics for suspect cases to be performed in appropriate BSL-3 laboratories with commercial NAATs and allow for routine laboratory investigations to be performed as point-of-care tests in relevant facilities, or in routine hospitals following discussions with local health authorities.[14]

Stand-alone, discrete analyzers may be used in high-level containment units either in combination with suited systems or in safety cabinets or isolators to protect staff. They are not recommended for use in routine hospital laboratories, are not considered to be safer than autoanalyzers, and should always be risk assessed.[10] A designated laboratory, adjacent to the patient facility at the HLIU at the Royal Free, uses small, POC analyzers to provide these supportive assays. POC analyzers and routine autoanalyzers may vary significantly in terms of performance. The benefits of POC analyzers, such as decreased size, portability, and ease of use, should be considered alongside the potentially poorer accuracy and precision of these assays. It is also important to remember that assay methodologies, and therefore normal ranges, vary between instruments. Therefore, results obtained on an autoanalyzer in a routine laboratory may not be directly comparable to the results obtained on POC instruments in a specialized center.

STAFF SAFETY

Recommendations are based on evidence from previously imported cases of VHF, settings where VHFs are endemic, and experience of laboratory-acquired infections. No recorded transmissions to laboratory workers were identified when reviewing previous imported cases of VHFs to resource-rich settings. In these cases, supportive assays had been performed using routine analyzers, in standard pathology laboratories, often before the diagnosis being made.[64–68] In addition, more than 9000 cases of CCHF were notified in the whole of Turkey (2002–2014), with an estimated minimum 180,000 blood samples processed in routine laboratories with no additional precautions. A review was performed of 51 health care exposures that occurred in 9 centers where 4869 of these patients were managed. Only 2 cases in laboratory staff were identified. One may have been associated with phlebotomy and the other with handling samples without appropriate personal protective equipment.[69] UK Health and Safety Executive data show that rates of infection with blood-borne viruses in health care workers are low, with the majority related to needle-stick injuries and not in laboratory staff.[70] Innumerable samples are processed daily in routine pathology laboratories that are, often unknown to us, positive for blood borne viruses. There is no evidence of any risk of transmission when good laboratory practice is followed within a Containment Level 2 laboratory.

Table 2
Summary of diagnostic antigen-based assays for Ebola virus disease

Company & Assay Name	Assay Target[a]	Performance[a]	Development Stage
Corgenix (Broomfield, CO, USA), ReEBOV Antigen Rapid Test	Lateral flow device for the detection of VP40 antigen in blood in approximately 20 min. The manufacturer has used the same technology for the detection of Lassa fever virus[72]	Blood sensitivity 100%, specificity 92.2%[73]	FDA approved. WHO approved for use in the detection of EVD where it is not possible to use a molecular assay
Chun-Yan Yen and colleagues' multiplexed lateral flow assay	Silver nanoparticles conjugated to detect EBOV GP (as well as Dengue and yellow fever viruses)[74]		Undergoing field studies; non commercial
France's Atomic Energy Commission (CEA, Paris, France) (with Vedalab, Cerisé, France) Ebola eZYSCREEN lateral flow assay	Handheld lateral flow device for the detection of EBOV antigens in blood, plasma, and urine <15 min		Commercially available
Stada Pharm (Bad Vilbel, Germany) and Senovas' (Weimar, Germany) Ebola lateral flow test	Handheld lateral flow device for the detection of EBOV antigens in blood and body fluids in 10 min		Commercially available
The UK's Defence Science and Technology Laboratory (Porton Down, UK) Ebola lateral flow assay	Semiquantitative detection of undisclosed EBOV antigen using capillary blood in 20 min	Blood sensitivity 100%, specificity 96.6%[75]	Not yet available
The US' Naval Medical Research Center (Silver Spring, MD, USA) Ebola lateral flow assay	Detection of undisclosed Ebola antigen using capillary blood in 15 min; can detect bola virus, Sudan virus, Taï Forest virus, and Reston virus	Blood sensitivity 87.8%, specificity 97.5% Oral swab sensitivity 88.9%, specificity 96.1%[76]	Not yet available

Abbreviation: VP40, viral protein 40.

[a] If available in published literature or from the manufacturer, all tested against Altona NAAT as gold standard.

INNOVATION IN EBOLA VIRUS DISEASE DIAGNOSTICS

The unprecedented scale and duration of the West Africa outbreak highlighted the paucity of diagnostics that are suited to the field. This lack of diagnostics resulted in the development of new technologies being offered for trial and approval[71] (see **Table 1**; **Table 2**). The location and setting of such outbreaks, together with them being sporadic and transient, suggest that simple POC assays would be of great benefit.[73] Several handheld lateral flow assays are being trialed and marketed currently, examples of which are detailed in **Table 2**. These assays detect viral antigens in blood and body fluids, require no electricity, can often be stored at ambient temperatures, and can provide a result within approximately 10 to 20 minutes. Given that many are reported to be highly sensitive, they may play a role as a negative screening tool. This attribute is of considerable importance given the likely need for repeated testing for suspected patients in the region.[75] It is desirable to be able to perform such tests on samples other than venous blood, for example, when appropriate venipuncture equipment is not available, or when confirming EVD as the cause of death in cadavers. In either case, it is safer for health care and public health staff to take oral swabs or finger-prick samples rather than to obtain venous blood samples and risk a sharps-related injury.[55,77] Achieving suitable regulatory approvals for new POC devices has, however, proved to be an obstacle to the rapid deployment of such assays, despite reported result times being available within 1 hour, excluding nucleic extraction.

Various rapid EBOV NAATs have been described, including reverse transcription-loop-mediated isothermal amplification (RT-LAMP),[55] other portable, low-cost, or handheld devices,[54,58] and the use of nanoparticles to detect isothermally amplified nucleic acids, shows promise.[57] It is clear that as equipment becomes more portable and data analysis becomes faster, it is likely that real-time genome sequencing of future outbreaks will bring real benefit in terms of epidemiology and monitoring viral variation. The feasibility of providing real-time genome sequencing in an outbreak setting has already been described.[78]

There is a continued need for investment in this area; new assays need to be developed, evaluated, and embedded into local health care systems to allow the prompt control of future outbreaks. Additional vigilance and surveillance are required to ensure that such assays meet the diagnostic needs as new viruses such as Bundibugyo Ebola virus are discovered[79] and inevitable sequence variation occurs.[80–83] Finally, up-skilling and investment in laboratory staff, along with sustained resourcing of basic pathology services, are fundamental for long-term resilience planning. The recent Ebola outbreak resulted in numerous lessons learned and significant innovation. As a result, it is hoped that future outbreaks will be identified faster and ultimately terminated more efficiently in part through greater access to portable, easy-to-use diagnostic assays.

Timely interruption of EVD transmission chains is vital for rapid control of future outbreaks, and novel strategies for doing so, including use of more localized testing, will likely play a key role in this. Lateral flow assays with high sensitivity and specificity may well be utilized in the United Kingdom and other resource-rich settings if repeat field testing is successful, in either specific EVD-diagnostic centers or even locally on blood draw of suspect patients.

SUMMARY

The 2014 to 2016 EVD, through the sheer size of the outbreak and combined experience within both resource-rich and resource-poor settings, allowed for more information to be gained in the clinical and pathologic features of EVD. This review has highlighted the range of aspects of EVD that the authors find are relevant to laboratory medicine, including the need for robust prediagnostic and laboratory processing algorithms to inform sampling of suspect patients, the vast majority of whom, in resource-rich settings, will have another diagnosis.

REFERENCES

1. Centers for Disease Control and Prevention. Outbreaks chronology: Ebola hemorrhagic fever [Internet]. Atlanta (GA): CDC; 2014. Available at: http://www.cdc.gov/vhf/ebola/resources/outbreak-table.html. Accessed September 6, 2016.

2. Kozak RA, Kobinger GP. Vaccines against "the other" Ebolavirus species. Expert Rev Vaccines 2016;15(9):1093–100.

3. World Health Organization. Statement on the 9th meeting of the IHR Emergency Committee regarding the Ebola outbreak in West Africa [Internet]. Geneva (Switzerland): WHO; 2016. Available at: http://www.who.int/mediacentre/news/statements/2016/end-of-ebola-pheic/en/. Accessed September 6, 2016.

4. World Health Organization. Ebola situation report—30 March 2016 [Internet]. Geneva (Switzerland): WHO; 2016. Available at: http://apps.who.int/ebola/current-situation/ebola-situation-report-30-march-2016. Accessed September 6, 2016.

5. Uyeki TM, Mehta AK, Davey RT, et al. Clinical management of Ebola virus disease in the United States and Europe. N Engl J Med 2016;374(7):636–46.

6. Gomes M, Pastore y Piontti A, Rossi L, et al. Assessing the international spreading risk associated with the 2014 West African ebola outbreak. PLoS Curr 2014. Available at: http://dx.doi.org/10.1371/currents.outbreaks.cd818f63d40e24aef769dda7df9e0da5. Accessed September 6, 2016.

7. Bogoch II, Creatore MI, Cetron MS, et al. Assessment of the potential for international dissemination of Ebola virus via commercial air travel during the 2014 west African outbreak. Lancet 2015;385(9962):29–35.

8. Read JM, Diggle PJ, Chirombo J, et al. Effectiveness of screening for Ebola at airports. Lancet 2015;385(9962):23–4.

9. Fletcher TE, Brooks TJG, Beeching NJ. Ebola and other viral haemorrhagic fevers. BMJ 2014;349:g5079.

10. Advisory Committee on Dangerous, Pathogens. Management of Hazard Group 4 viral haemorrhagic fevers and similar human infectious diseases of high consequence. Advisory Committee on Dangerous Pathogens [Internet]. London: ACDP; 2015. Available at: https://www.gov.uk/government/uploads/system/uploads/attachment_data/file/534002/Management_of_VHF_A.pdf. Accessed September 6, 2016.

11. Public Health England. Imported fever service (IFS) [Internet]. London: PHE; 2014. Available at: https://www.gov.uk/guidance/imported-fever-service-ifs. Accessed September 6, 2016.

12. Centers for Disease Control and Prevention. Notes on the Interim U.S. Guidance for monitoring and movement of persons with potential Ebola virus exposure [Internet]. Atlanta (GA): CDC; 2016. Available at: http://www.cdc.gov/vhf/ebola/exposure/monitoring-and-movement-of-persons-with-exposure.html. Accessed September 6, 2016.

13. Centers for Disease Control and Prevention. Epidemiologic risk factors to consider when evaluating a person for exposure to Ebola virus [Internet]. Atlanta (GA): CDC; 2015. Available at: http://www.cdc.gov/vhf/ebola/exposure/risk-factors-when-evaluating-person-for-exposure.html. Accessed September 6, 2016.

14. Robert Koch Institute. Framework Ebola virus disease (3rd update) [Internet]. Berlin: RKI; 2016. Available at: http://www.rki.de/EN/Content/infections/

epidemiology/outbreaks/Ebola_virus_disease/Framework_EVD.html. Accessed September 6, 2016.

15. The College of Emergency Medicine & Public Health England. Best practice guideline—Ebola guidance for emergency departments [Internet]. London: CEM; 2016. Available at: www.rcem.ac.uk/CEM/document?id=805. Accessed September 6, 2016.

16. Centers for Disease Control and Prevention. Interim guidance for U.S. Hospital preparedness for patients under investigation (PUIs) or with confirmed Ebola virus disease (EVD): a framework for a tiered approach [Internet]. Atlanta (GA): CDC; 2015. Available at: http://www.cdc.gov/vhf/ebola/healthcare-us/preparing/hospitals.html. Accessed September 6, 2016.

17. Ergönül O. Crimean-Congo haemorrhagic fever. Lancet Infect Dis 2006;6(4): 203–14.

18. Leligdowicz A, Fischer WA, Uyeki TM, et al. Ebola virus disease and critical illness. Crit Care 2016;20(1):217.

19. Chertow DS, Kleine C, Edwards JK, et al. Ebola virus disease in West Africa–clinical manifestations and management. N Engl J Med 2014;371(22):2054–7.

20. Lado M, Walker NF, Baker P, et al. Clinical features of patients isolated for suspected Ebola virus disease at Connaught Hospital, Freetown, Sierra Leone: a retrospective cohort study. Lancet Infect Dis 2015;15(9):1024–33.

21. Dallatomasina S, Crestani R, Sylvester Squire J, et al. Ebola outbreak in rural West Africa: epidemiology, clinical features and outcomes. Trop Med Int Health 2015;20(4):448–54.

22. Arranz J, Lundeby KM, Hassan S, et al. Clinical features of suspected Ebola cases referred to the Moyamba ETC, Sierra Leone: challenges in the later stages of the 2014 outbreak. BMC Infect Dis 2016;16:308.

23. Levine AC, Shetty PP, Burbach R, et al. Derivation and internal validation of the Ebola prediction score for risk stratification of patients with suspected Ebola virus disease. Ann Emerg Med 2015;66(3):285–93.e1.

24. Yan T, Mu J, Qin E, et al. Clinical characteristics of 154 patients suspected of having Ebola virus disease in the Ebola holding center of Jui Government Hospital in Sierra Leone during the 2014 Ebola outbreak. Eur J Clin Microbiol Infect Dis 2015; 34(10):2089–95.

25. Fitzgerald F, Awonuga W, Shah T, et al. Ebola response in Sierra Leone: the impact on children. J Infect 2016;72(Suppl):S6–12.

26. Shah T, Greig J, van der Plas LM, et al. Inpatient signs and symptoms and factors associated with death in children aged 5 years and younger admitted to two Ebola management centres in Sierra Leone, 2014: a retrospective cohort study. Lancet Glob Heal 2016;4(7):e495–501.

27. Scott JT, Sesay FR, Massaquoi TA, et al. Post-Ebola syndrome, Sierra Leone. Emerg Infect Dis 2016;22(4):641–6.

28. Tiffany A, Vetter P, Mattia J, et al. Ebola virus disease complications as experienced by survivors in Sierra Leone. Clin Infect Dis 2016;62(11):1360–6.

29. Mattia JG, Vandy MJ, Chang JC, et al. Early clinical sequelae of Ebola virus disease in Sierra Leone: a cross-sectional study. Lancet Infect Dis 2016;16(3):331–8.

30. Vetter P, Kaiser L, Schibler M, et al. Sequelae of Ebola virus disease: the emergency within the emergency. Lancet Infect Dis 2016;16(6):e82–91.

31. Howlett P, Brown C, Helderman T, et al. Ebola virus disease complicated by late-onset encephalitis and polyarthritis, Sierra Leone. Emerg Infect Dis 2016;22(1):150–2.

32. Jacobs M, Rodger A, Bell DJ, et al. Late Ebola virus relapse causing meningoencephalitis: a case report. Lancet 2016;388(10043):498–503.

33. Varkey JB, Shantha JG, Crozier I, et al. Persistence of ebola virus in ocular fluid during convalescence. N Engl J Med 2015;372(25):2423–7.

34. Akerlund E, Prescott J, Tampellini L. Shedding of ebola virus in an asymptomatic pregnant woman. N Engl J Med 2015;372(25):2467–9.

35. Dean NE, Halloran ME, Yang Y, et al. Transmissibility and pathogenicity of Ebola virus: a systematic review and meta-analysis of household secondary attack rate and asymptomatic infection. Clin Infect Dis 2016;62(10):1277–86.

36. Thorson A, Formenty P, Lofthouse C, et al. Systematic review of the literature on viral persistence and sexual transmission from recovered Ebola survivors: evidence and recommendations. BMJ Open 2016;6(1):e008859.

37. Diallo B, Sissoko D, Loman NJ, et al. Resurgence of Ebola virus disease in Guinea linked to a survivor with virus persistence in seminal fluid for more than 500 days. Clin Infect Dis 2016;63(10):1353–6.

38. Chughtai AA, Barnes M, Macintyre CR. Persistence of Ebola virus in various body fluids during convalescence: evidence and implications for disease transmission and control. Epidemiol Infect 2016;144(8):1652–60.

39. Green E, Hunt L, Ross JCG, et al. Viraemia and Ebola virus secretion in survivors of Ebola virus disease in Sierra Leone: a cross-sectional cohort study. Lancet Infect Dis 2016;16(9):1052–6.

40. Hunt L, Gupta-Wright A, Simms V, et al. Clinical presentation, biochemical, and haematological parameters and their association with outcome in patients with Ebola virus disease: an observational cohort study. Lancet Infect Dis 2015; 15(11):1292–9.

41. Kortepeter MG, Bausch DG, Bray M. Basic clinical and laboratory features of filoviral hemorrhagic fever. J Infect Dis 2011;204:S810–6.

42. Moole H, Chitta S, Victor D, et al. Association of clinical signs and symptoms of Ebola viral disease with case fatality: a systematic review and meta-analysis. J Community Hosp Intern Med Perspect 2015;5(4):28406.

43. Zhang X, Rong Y, Sun L, et al. Prognostic analysis of patients with ebola virus disease. PLoS Negl Trop Dis 2015;9(9):e0004113.

44. Qin E, Bi J, Zhao M, et al. Clinical features of patients with Ebola virus disease in Sierra Leone. Clin Infect Dis 2015;61(4):491–5.

45. Barry M, Traoré FA, Sako FB, et al. Ebola outbreak in Conakry, Guinea: epidemiological, clinical, and outcome features. Med Mal Infect 2014;44(11–12):491–4.

46. Li J, Duan H-J, Chen H-Y, et al. Age and Ebola viral load correlate with mortality and survival time in 288 Ebola virus disease patients. Int J Infect Dis 2016;42: 34–9.

47. Fitzpatrick G, Vogt F, Moi Gbabai OB, et al. The contribution of Ebola viral load at admission and other patient characteristics to mortality in a Médecins Sans Frontières Ebola Case Management Centre, Kailahun, Sierra Leone, June-October 2014. J Infect Dis 2015;212(11):1752–8.

48. Schieffelin JS, Shaffer JG, Goba A, Gbakie M, Gire SK, Colubri A, et al. Clinical illness and outcomes in patients with Ebola in Sierra Leone. N Engl J Med 2014;371(22):2092–100.

49. Akinci E, Bodur H, Sunbul M, et al. Prognostic factors, pathophysiology and novel biomarkers in Crimean-Congo hemorrhagic fever. Antiviral Res 2016;132:233–43.

50. Cherpillod P, Schibler M, Vieille G, et al. Ebola virus disease diagnosis by real-time RT-PCR: a comparative study of 11 different procedures. J Clin Virol 2016; 77:9–14.

51. Southern TR, Racsa LD, Albario CG, et al. Comparison of FilmArray and quantitative real-time reverse transcriptase PCR for detection of Zaire Ebolavirus from contrived and clinical specimens. J Clin Microbiol 2015;53(9):2956–60.

52. Leski T, Ansumana R, Taitt CR, et al. Use of the FilmArray system for detection of Zaire ebolavirus in a small hospital in Bo, Sierra Leone. J Clin Microbiol 2015; 53(7):2368–70.

53. Pinsky B, Sahoo MK, Sandlund J, et al. Analytical performance characteristics of the cepheid GeneXpert Ebola Assay for the detection of Ebola virus. PLoS One 2015;10(11):1–16.

54. Ahrberg CD, Manz A, Neuzil P. Palm-sized device for point-of-care Ebola detection. Anal Chem 2016;88(9):4803–7.

55. Kurosaki Y, Magassouba N, Oloniniyi OK, et al. Development and evaluation of reverse transcription-loop-mediated isothermal amplification (RT-LAMP) assay coupled with a portable device for rapid diagnosis of Ebola virus disease in Guinea. Plos Negl Trop Dis 2016;10(2):1–12.

56. Panning M, Laue T, Olschlager S, et al. Diagnostic reverse-transcription polymerase chain reaction kit for filoviruses based on the strain collections of all European biosafety level 4 laboratories. J Infect Dis 2007;196(Suppl):S199–204.

57. Wang Y, Zhu G, Qi W, et al. A versatile quantitation platform based on platinum nanoparticles incorporated volumetric bar-chart chip for highly sensitive assays. Biosens Bioelectron 2016;85:777–84.

58. Chan K, Wong PY, Yu P, et al. A rapid and low-cost PCR thermal cycler for infectious disease diagnostics. PLoS One 2016;11(2):1–17.

59. Trombley AR, Wachter L, Garrison J, et al. Short report: comprehensive panel of real-time TaqMan polymerase chain reaction assays for detection and absolute quantification of filoviruses, arenaviruses, and new world hantaviruses. Am J Trop Med Hyg 2010;82(5):954–60.

60. US Department of Health and Human Services Public Health Service. Centers for Disease Control & Prevention, and National Institutes of Health. Biosafety in microbiological and biomedical laboratories. 5th edition. Atlanta (GA): CDC; 1999.

61. Centers for Disease Control and Prevention (CDC). Hospital preparedness: a tiered approach [Internet]. Atlanta (GA): CDC; 2015. Available at: http://www.cdc.gov/vhf/ebola/healthcare-us/preparing/treatment-centers.html. Accessed September 6, 2016.

62. Department of Health. Environment and sustainability Health Technical Memorandum 07-01: safe management of healthcare waste. London: DH; 2013.

63. Centers for Disease Control and Prevention and World Health Organization. Guidance for collection, transport and submission of specimens for Ebola virus testing [Internet]. Atlanta (GA): CDC; 2015. Available at: http://www.cdc.gov/vhf/ebola/healthcare-us/laboratories/specimens.html. Accessed September 6, 2016.

64. Crowcroft NS, Meltzer M, Evans M, et al. The public health response to a case of Lassa fever in London in 2000. J Infect 2004;48(3):221–8.

65. Atkin S, Anaraki S, Gothard P, et al. The first case of Lassa fever imported from Mali to the United Kingdom, February 2009. Euro Surveill 2009;14(10):2–4.

66. Kitching A, Addiman S, Cathcart S, et al. A fatal case of Lassa fever in London, January 2009. Euro Surveill 2009;14(6):2–4.

67. Haas WH, Breuer T, Pfaff G, et al. Imported Lassa fever in Germany: surveillance and management of contact persons. Clin Infect Dis 2003;36(10):1254–8.

68. Barr DA, Aitken C, Bell DJ, et al. First confirmed case of Crimean-Congo haemorrhagic fever in the UK. Lancet 2013;382(9902):1458.

69. Leblebicioglu H, Sunbul M, Guner R, et al. Healthcare-associated Crimean-Congo haemorrhagic fever in Turkey, 2002-2014: a multicentre retrospective cross-sectional study. Clin Microbiol Infect 2016;22(4):387.e1-4.
70. Public Health England. Bloodborne viruses: eye of the needle [Internet]. London: PHE; 2014. Available at: https://www.gov.uk/government/publications/bloodborne-viruses-eye-of-the-needle. Accessed September 6, 2016.
71. Butler D. Ebola experts seek to expand testing. Nature 2014;516(7530):154–5.
72. Boisen ML, Schieffelin JS, Goba A, et al. Multiple circulating infections can mimic the early stages of viral hemorrhagic fevers and possible human exposure to filoviruses in Sierra Leone prior to the 2014 outbreak. Viral Immunol 2015;28(1): 19–31.
73. Broadhurst MJ, Kelly JD, Miller A, et al. ReEBOV Antigen Rapid Test kit for point-of-care and laboratory-based testing for Ebola virus disease: a field validation study. Lancet 2015;6736(15):1–8.
74. Yen C-W, de Puig H, Tam JO, et al. Multicolored silver nanoparticles for multiplexed disease diagnostics: distinguishing dengue, yellow fever, and Ebola viruses. Lab Chip 2015;15:1638–41.
75. Walker NF, Brown CS, Youkee D, et al. Evaluation of a point-of-care blood test for identification of Ebola virus disease at Ebola holding units, Western Area, Sierra Leone, January to February 2015. Euro Surveill 2015;20(12):1–6.
76. Phan JC, Pettitt J, George JS, et al. Lateral flow immunoassays for ebola virus disease detection in Liberia. J Infect Dis 2016;214(suppl 3):S222–8.
77. Formenty P, Leroy EM, Epelboin A, et al. Detection of Ebola virus in oral fluid specimens during outbreaks of Ebola virus hemorrhagic fever in the Republic of Congo. Clin Infect Dis 2006;42(11):1521–6.
78. Quick J, Loman NJ, Duraffour S, et al. Real-time, portable genome sequencing for Ebola surveillance. Nature 2016;530(7589):228–32.
79. Towner JS, Sealy TK, Khristova ML, et al. Newly discovered Ebola virus associated with hemorrhagic fever outbreak in Uganda. PLoS Pathog 2008;4(11):3–8.
80. Carroll SA, Towner JS, Sealy TK, et al. Molecular evolution of viruses of the family Filoviridae based on 97 whole-genome sequences. J Virol 2013;87(5):2608–16.
81. Carroll MW, Matthews DA, Elmore MJ, et al. Temporal and spatial analysis of the 2014–2015 Ebola virus outbreak in West Africa. Nature 2015;524(7563):97–101.
82. Gire SK, Goba A, Andersen KG, et al. Genomic surveillance elucidates Ebola virus origin and transmission during the 2014 outbreak. Science 2014;345(6202): 1369–72.
83. Hoenen T, Safronetz D, Groseth A, et al. Mutation rate and genotype variation of Ebola virus from Mali case sequences. Science 2015;348(6230):117–9.

Rift Valley Fever

 CrossMark

Amy Hartman, PhD

KEYWORDS

- Rift Valley fever • Mosquitos • Transmission • Treatment

KEY POINTS

- Rift Valley fever (RVF) is an important human and veterinary pathogen that causes significant illness and death.
- The life cycle of RVF is complex and involves mosquitoes, livestock, climate, and humans.
- RVF virus is transmitted from either mosquitoes or animals to humans, but is generally not transmitted from person to person.
- There is a significant risk of emergence of RVF into new locations, which would affect human health and livestock industries.
- There are no approved vaccines or therapeutics to treat human RVF.

OVERVIEW

One Health is a concept that recognizes the inextricable linkages between human health, animal health, and the environment (**Fig. 1**). Rift Valley fever (RVF) is a long-recognized veterinary disease of livestock in Africa. Infection with RVF virus (RVFV) causes a highly lethal illness in domesticated livestock (sheep, cattle, and goats) that consequently has dire economic impacts in affected regions. RVF has been and remains on the World Organization for Animal Health's list of notifiable animal diseases of concern.[1] Mosquitoes serve as both the reservoir and vector for RVFV. Because mosquito breeding depends on rainfall, the occurrences of RVF outbreaks are linked to environmental conditions and thus are likely to be affected by climate change. Epizootic spillover to humans occurs by both mosquito bite and from direct handling of infected animal carcasses.

The geographic distribution of RVF has broadened since its discovery in 1931.[2] Initially a disease of the Rift Valley in eastern Africa, RVF has emerged throughout continental Africa as well as in Madagascar and the Saudi Arabian peninsula. Importantly, the insect vectors that transmit RVFV are found in Europe and the Americas, which opens the door to emergence in new locations and could cause considerable human morbidity and mortality as well as economic damage.[3–6] The introduction and rapid spread of West Nile Virus into the United States in the last 17 years (and Chikungunya

Center for Vaccine Research, Infectious Diseases and Microbiology, University of Pittsburgh Graduate School of Public Health, University of Pittsburgh, 3501 Fifth Avenue, Pittsburgh, PA 15260, USA
E-mail address: hartman2@pitt.edu

Clin Lab Med 37 (2017) 285–301
http://dx.doi.org/10.1016/j.cll.2017.01.004
0272-2712/17/© 2017 Elsevier Inc. All rights reserved.
labmed.theclinics.com

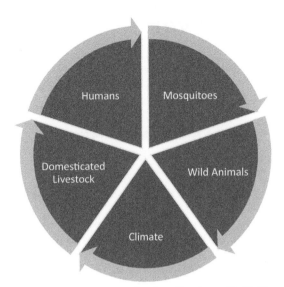

Fig. 1. Important players in the ecology of Rift Valley fever (RVF). The dynamics of RVF depend on the complex interplay between humans, mosquitoes, wild and domesticated animals, and the environment.

and Zika viruses more recently) serves as a good barometer for the impact of importation of another mosquito-borne virus such as RVFV. In addition to its potential as an emerging viral disease, RVFV is listed as a National Institute of Allergy and Infectious Disease category A priority pathogen, is on the list of federal Select Agents and Toxins, and is considered a potential bioterror threat owing to the ease of infection by inhalation.[7,8]

In 2015, the World Health Organization's Workshop on Prioritization of Pathogens assigned RVF to the list of "severe emerging diseases with potential to generate a public health emergency, and for which no, or insufficient, preventive and curative solutions exist."[9] This group of experts recommended urgent research and development to address this need. At the same time, *Science* magazine listed RVF on the top 10 list of high priorities for research based on the need for vaccines and therapeutics.[10] Thus, RVF is clearly a relevant emerging disease that could cause considerable economic damage and human morbidity and mortality if it emerged in new locations. This review article examines the epidemiology and clinical profile of RVF.

MICROBIOLOGY

RVFV is one of the most important members of the large and diverse *Bunyaviridae* family. RVFV belongs to the *Phlebovirus* genus, which also contains other viruses including Punta Toro, Sandfly fever, and severe fever with thrombocytopenia syndrome virus. The name phleobovirus is derived from the fact that most of the viruses in this genus are transmitted by phlebotomine sandflies. RVFV is a notable exception because it is transmitted primarily by mosquitoes. All bunyaviruses, including RVFV, contain a tripartite genome consisting of 3 single-stranded, negative-polarity RNA segments. The genome segments are creatively named large (L), medium (M), and small (S). The L segment encodes the viral polymerase protein. The M segment encodes the glycoproteins (Gn and Gc), as well as a nonstructural protein termed

NSm. Both L and M segments use a negative-sense coding strategy. In contrast, some phleboviruses such as RVFV use an ambisense coding strategy for the S segment. The nucleoprotein (N) is encoded with negative polarity on the S segment, whereas a second nonstructural protein, NSs, is encoded with positive polarity. Nucleocapsids consist of the viral nucleoprotein (N) multiplexed with each RNA segment. Complementary nucleotide sequences at the 3' and 5' ends of each segment are thought to form circular RNAs.[11,12]

Cells become infected with RVFV by receptor-mediated endocytosis, followed by pH-mediated fusion of virus endosomal membranes to release nucleocapsids into the cell cytoplasm. Transcription, translation, and genome replication occur in the cytoplasm. A unique aspect to the life cycle of RVFV and other bunyaviruses is that mature viral particles assemble and bud from the Golgi apparatus in some cell types.[13]

Genomic sequence analysis of RVFV strains obtained between 1944 and 2007 reveal relatively low (5%) sequence divergence.[14,15] There are at least 7 genetic lineages, yet lineage does not correlate with geographic origin, indicating that there is substantial regional movement of genotypes. Genetic evidence exists for the reassortment of viral segments in nature but no indication of recombination.[15,16]

EPIDEMIOLOGY

The epidemiology of RVFV is complex and involves multiple players, including mosquitoes, wild animals, domesticated livestock, and humans (**Fig. 2**).

Mosquitoes

RVFV has been isolated from a wide range of mosquito species spanning several genera (**Table 1**). *Aedes* mosquitoes are the primary reservoir and vector, although *Culex*, *Anopheles*, and *Mansonia* are important secondary vectors that contribute to amplification of epizootics and epidemics.[17,18] The virus has also been isolated from other mosquito genera, as well as ticks, flies, and midges,[19–21] but their role in biological transmission is unknown.

A unique aspect to the biology of RVFV is that the virus is maintained by transovarial transmission within *Aedes* mosquito eggs, meaning that live virus can be passed from parent mosquito to offspring by maintenance within eggs[22] (see **Fig. 2**). During interepidemic periods, the virus remains infectious within dormant desiccated *Aedes* mosquito eggs in dry floodplains; infected mosquitoes will emerge during flooding. As would be expected, outbreaks are associated with unusually heavy rainfall, especially cyclical *El Nino*–southern oscillation weather patterns.[23]

Mammals

Like most arboviruses, RVFV alternates between mosquitoes and vertebrate hosts. Evidence of RVFV infection (as determined by hemagglutinin inhibition or plaque-reducing neutralizing antibody titers) has been found in many wild mammalian species in Africa, including camels, bats, lions, and elephants (**Table 2**).[24–26] The virus causes mild or inapparent illness in these species. It is not known whether any of the wild animal species are amplifying hosts.

Unlike wild animals, RVFV is highly pathogenic in domesticated ruminants, which are the amplifying hosts, meaning that they develop sufficient viremia to infect feeding mosquitoes and potentiate further transmission. The most severe disease occurs in developing fetuses and very young animals immediately after birth; older animals are somewhat more resistant. A description of disease in the 3 most common domestic animals (cattle, sheep, and goats) is summarized in **Table 3**. High titers of virus are

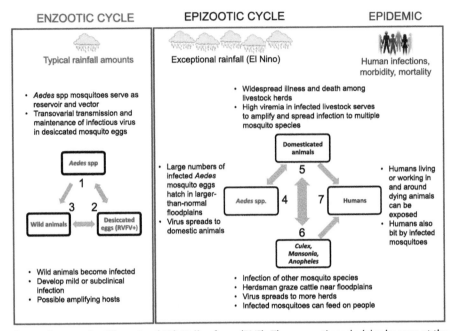

Fig. 2. The complex life cycle of Rift Valley fever (RVF). The enzootic cycle (also known at the sylvatic or cryptic cycle; *green*) occurs under normal rainfall conditions. Infected *Aedes* mosquitoes serve as both the reservoir and vector (#1). Infectious virus can survive for years in desiccated mosquito eggs (#2). Normal rainfall leads to formation of small floodplains (dambos), in which the infected mosquito eggs hatch. Infected adult mosquitoes will then feed on and infect wild ungulates (#3); their role in transmission cycle is not well understood. Heavy rainfall conditions, such as *El Nino*–southern oscillation events, can lead to the epizootic cycle (also known as the domestic cycle; *blue*). Larger flood plains increase the likelihood of interaction between domesticated livestock and mosquitoes (#4,5), resulting in illness, abortion, and death. Other species of mosquito (*Culex, Anopheles*) can feed off of viremic animals and transfer the virus longer distances and to other herds (#6). Human epidemics occur when there are many infected and dying animals. People can be infected by mosquito or by handling infected animals (#7).

Table 1	
Insect genera and potential role in life cycle of Rift Valley fever	
Genus	**Type of Vector**
Aedes	Primary enzootic reservoir and vector
Culex	Secondary vector
Mansonia	Secondary vector
Anopheles	Secondary vector
Coquillettidia	Secondary vector
Eretmapodites	Secondary vector
Culicoides (biting midges)	Role unknown
Plebotomus (sand flies)	Role unknown
Simulium (other flies)	Role unknown

Data from Refs.[17–21]

Table 2	
Wild and domesticated animals with evidence of Rift Valley fever infection	
Susceptible Wild Animals[a]	**Domesticated Animals[b]**
Springbok	Cattle
Wildebeest	Sheep
Impala	Goats
Lions	Buffalo
Gazelles	Camels
African buffalo	Horses
Warthogs	Donkeys
Elephants	
Bats	
Rhinocerous	
Murine rodents	

[a] Based on detection of neutralizing antibodies or hemagglutinin inhibition.
[b] Susceptible to disease.
Data from Refs.[24–26,109]

found in the blood of infected animals for approximately a week after onset of illness. Direct animal-to-animal transmission of RVFV does not occur among herds nor experimentally in the laboratory. *Culex* and *Mansonia* mosquitoes are thought to be responsible for horizontal transmission between viremic animals and humans (see **Fig. 2**).[27]

Humans

Humans become infected with RVFV when there is widespread illness and death among domesticated livestock. People can be infected by the bite of a mosquito, but the primary means of transmission of the virus to people is thought to be through mucous membrane exposure or inhalation of viral particles during the handling of infected animals and carcasses. A number of retrospective studies suggest that touching/ handling, living close to, and consuming animal products are factors associated with increased likelihood of RVFV infection and possibly more severe outcomes.[21,28–32] Between 1997 and 2010, there were 9 RVFV outbreaks, with 1220 confirmed human deaths and more than 500,000 estimated human cases.[33] Most recently in March of 2016, human cases of RVF, associated with an outbreak in goats, occurred in Uganda.[34] One of these patients was a butcher, and the other reported to have interacted with sick animals.[35] The virus has not shown direct human-to-human transmission, and there have been only a few documented cases of vertical transmission.[36–38]

BIOSAFETY AND BIODEFENSE CONCERNS

Of note, a significant number of accidental infections with RVFV have occurred among people performing diagnostic testing or those working with the virus in animals or the laboratory.[39–43] At least 25 accidental infections occurred through 1949,[39] with a total of 47 to date. Many of these infections were traced to aerosol (inhalational) exposure.[39,40] These laboratory-acquired infections led to early knowledge about the disease course in humans.

The United States, Canada, Japan, the former Soviet Union, and potentially other nations performed research on RVFV within their offensive biological weapons programs during the height of the Cold War.[44–51] Mention of RVFV dates back to the origin of the United States offensive program in 1941 with the establishment of the Bacteriologic Warfare Committee.[52]

Table 3
Rift Valley fever disease in domesticated animals

	Adult Sheep or Goats	Lambs or Kids	Adult Cattle	Calves
Peracute disease?	Yes	No	Yes	No
Acute clinical disease	Fever, weakness, anorexia, diarrhea, bloody nasal discharge, jaundice, increased respiration; leukopenia, elevated liver enzymes, jaundice	High fever, listlessness, inactivity, anorexia; abdominal pain; increased respiration rate; bleeding and hemorrhage from the ruminant stomach; blood in intestine	Weakness, anorexia, bloody diarrhea, hypersalivation, bloody nasal discharge	Jaundice, fever, weakness, anorexia, bloody diarrhea
Macroscopic pathology	Liver seems to be mottled owing to cell necrosis and hemorrhage; enlarged lymph nodes	Enlarged, friable liver (mottled owing to necrotic foci and hemorrhage); spleen: capsular hemorrhage with some enlargement; enlarged lymph nodes	Liver seems to be mottled owing to cell necrosis and hemorrhage; enlarged lymph nodes	Enlarged, friable liver; enlarged spleen with some hemorrhage; enlarged lymph nodes
Microscopic pathology	Hepatic and splenic necrosis (less severe and extensive than lambs)	Hepatic necrosis; lung congestion; hemorrhage in mucosa of abomasum; necrosis of spleen; pyknotic/karyorrhexic kidney; sporadic necrosis in small intestine	Hepatic and splenic necrosis (less severe and extensive than calves)	Hepatic and splenic necrosis; lung congestion
Time frame	3 d	<36 h	2–3 d	2–8 d
Mortality rate (%)	30–50	90	5–10	20
Fetal effects	Frequent abortion (up to 100%)	—	Comparatively less frequent abortion (up to 85%)	—

Data from Refs. 2,58,59,96,110–112

Although much of the information concerning the United States' bioweapon program is still classified, records indicate that research on RVF was conducted under Operation Whitecoat, which was the primary US biodefense medical research program between 1954 and 1973.[53,54] In 1968 and 1969, a formalin-inactivated vaccine against RVF (termed NDBR 103 RVFV) was tested in volunteers under approved clinical protocols; the vaccine provided enough protection to receive investigational new drug status from the Food and Drug Administration. Volunteers were likely exposed to RVFV, presumably by aerosol, although further details about the specifics of the human testing with RVFV have not been declassified to date. This research concluded when President Richard M. Nixon ended the offensive biological weapon program in 1969 and the United States signed the Biological Weapons Convention in 1972. Despite its history, there are conflicting opinions on the current likelihood of the use of RVFV as a bioweapon.[33,55]

Because RVF can be acquired through inhalation, RVFV is classified as a Risk Group 3 agent, and biosafety level 3 containment requirements are needed to work with the virus in the laboratory.[56] It is also a Select Agent that is regulated by both the Centers for Disease Control and Prevention and US Department of Agriculture/Animal and Plant Health Inspection Service.[7,8]

CLINICAL PRESENTATION
Livestock

The clinical disease of RVF in domesticated animals is described in **Table 3**.[2,57–59] At all stages of gestation, infection of pregnant domesticated animals will result in near 100% death of the fetuses. Adult livestock are susceptible to peracute disease, which is defined as the occurrence of death before the development of any clinical signs. Adult livestock can also develop acute disease characterized by weakness, anorexia, diarrhea, bloody nasal discharge, and jaundice. The mortality rate depends on the species and age of the animal, with sheep and goats generally being more susceptible to death than cattle (see **Table 3**). In livestock, the liver is the primary target of the virus, and characteristic lesions of RVF include widespread areas of necrosis and hemorrhage, giving the liver a mottled appearance. More extensive liver lesions are associated with more severe disease. Necrosis and hemorrhage are also seen in the splenic pulp. Hemorrhage and blood in the stomach and small intestine can lead to bloody diarrhea.

Humans

Most infected people develop uncomplicated RVF, which is characterized by nonspecific flulike symptoms with fever[60] (**Table 4**). In some patients, a biphasic fever occurs (3 days of fever, 1–2 days of remission, followed by another 2–3 days of fever).[31] Although this is not lethal, symptoms can be debilitating, and convalescence may take several weeks.

However, there are 3 additional more severe clinical outcomes that occur in some people infected with RVFV (see **Table 4**). Ocular complications are the most frequently reported (up to 10% of infected people).[31,61–64] Patients have reduced vision (either bilateral or unilateral), blind or black spots, photophobia, and retroorbital pain. Examination reveals inflammation of the retina and vessels of the eye, including retinal hemorrhage. Vision defects are not always permanent and may take weeks to months to resolve.

A severe hepatotropic disease (similar to that seen in sheep and other domesticated animals) occurs in people at an estimated frequency of about 1% to 2%. In addition to

Table 4
Human clinical symptoms of Rift Valley fever

Uncomplicated	Ocular Complications	Hemorrhagic Complications	Meningoencephalitis
Headache	Vision reduction	Jaundice	Severe headache
Body aches	Blind spots	Blood in urine/feces	Hallucination
Fever	Photophobia	Vomiting blood	Disorientation
Abdominal pain	Retroorbital pain	Purple rash	Vertigo
Joint/muscle aches	Uveitis	Gingival bleeding	Excessive salivation
Vomiting	Retinitis		Weakness
Anorexia			Partial paralysis
Weakness			
Nosebleeds			
Sweating			
Constipation			

Data from Refs.[21,30–32,60–65]

the nonspecific symptoms described, these patients also develop jaundice and hemorrhagic manifestations (blood in urine/feces, vomiting of blood, purple skin rash, gingival bleeding).[60] Evidence of liver necrosis is seen on autopsy, and prolonged blood coagulation times are noted.[21,65]

The third complication that can arise in RVF patients is neurologic disease, typically with a delayed onset. The delay can be anywhere from 5 to 30 days after the initial febrile illness. Clinical signs include severe headache, hallucination, disorientation, vertigo, excessive salivation, and weakness or partial paralysis.[21,30,32] This form of RVF can be lethal (53% of patients with neurologic complications died during the 2000 Saudi outbreak); in survivors, symptoms may be prolonged and even permanent.[30]

Mechanisms determining the different disease outcomes in humans are not understood fully, but there is recent evidence that genetic polymorphisms, coinfections, and comorbidities may contribute to more severe disease outcomes.[28,66,67] Even though isolated cases of vertical transmission have been documented,[36–38] there seems to be no increase in apparent miscarriage in pregnant women. There is also no documented human-to-human transmission; infection of people seems to be limited to either mosquito bites or exposure to high titer animal tissues. Despite this, viral RNA was detected by polymerase chain reaction in urine and semen from an immunosuppressed transplant recipient 4 months after illness.[68] It is not known what role (if any) this may play in transmission and spread.

DIAGNOSIS

In endemic regions, human illness soon follows in areas where there is concurrent RVF disease in animals, so monitoring of herds and efficient reporting is critical. Blood samples from acutely infected people can be tested for the presence of virus by either reverse transcriptase polymerase chain reaction, antigen-detection enzyme-linked immunosorbent assay, or isolation of live virus. After the cessation of viremia, immunoglobulin (Ig)M can be detected transiently. Recovered patients will have persistent IgG antibodies for years after infection, and thus can be useful for determining seropositivity and historical infection rates. Although some rapid diagnostic tests are in development, none are available yet commercially. Currently, the availability of clinical testing is only though international reference laboratories such as the Centers for Disease Control and Prevention in Atlanta, Georgia, the Kenya Medical Research Institute, and the Onderstepoort Veterinary Institute in South Africa, among others.[69]

TREATMENT AND PREVENTION

There are no specific, Food and Drug Administration-approved treatments for RVF. Treatment of symptoms such as fever and body aches can be done with standard over-the-counter medications. Care of hospitalized patients is supportive, including fluid replacement. Drugs that affect the liver, kidney, or coagulation should be avoided.

Therapeutics

Historically, ribavirin has been looked to as a potential antiviral therapeutic for RVF because of its demonstrated in vitro efficacy, and it has some limited in vivo efficacy against other emerging hemorrhagic fever viruses (Lassa fever, Crimean-Congo hemorrhagic fever).[70–72] However, intravenous administration of ribavirin to patients during the 2000 outbreak in Saudi Arabia was quickly stopped owing the finding that it may increase the likelihood of neurologic disease.[73] Newer broad-spectrum antiviral drugs such as favipiravir have shown some promise in rodent models.[74]

Vaccines

RVF presents a unique opportunity to merge facets of both veterinary and human vaccination strategies under the One Health concept. Vaccination of livestock will not only help to control epizootics but also prevent the chain of transmission to humans (reviewed in Ref.[75]). Since the 1960s, formalin-inactivated vaccines have been used to protect laboratory workers from accidental exposure. The NDBR 103 vaccine was arguably one of the biggest successes of the Operation Whitecoat program. After the initial clinical trials, the vaccine was used for years to vaccinate and protect laboratory workers. The ultimate test came during the 1977 outbreak in Egypt where the highly virulent ZH501 strain emerged to cause lethal disease in people. US naval soldiers working with the virus from patient samples at Naval Medical Research Unit No. 3 (NAMRU-3) off the coast of Egypt were given the NDBR 103 experimental vaccine. Since then, a next-generation version of a formalin inactivated vaccine, TSI GSD 200, has been used to vaccinate laboratory workers and high-risk personnel to this day through the Special Immunizations Program.[76]

A significant drawback of the formalin-inactivated vaccine is that the development of an adequate immune response requires 3 inoculations, making this impractical for use in livestock.[77–79] To overcome this, several live-attenuated vaccines, such as MP-12 and Clone 13, were generated and tested in the 1980s and 1990s.[80] Protection of experimentally inoculated animals from virulent challenge was achieved, but there is a potential for teratogenic effects in pregnant animals.[81–84] Another disadvantage is that use of live-attenuated RVF vaccines during epizootics have shown the potential for reversion to virulence and spread from animal to animal.[85] Despite these potential limitations, MP-12 is still being pursued as a human vaccine to this day.[86–88]

More recently, reverse genetics has allowed generation of rationally designed live attenuated vaccines. A recombinant virus with deletions in the NSs and NSm proteins (termed ZH501-ΔNSs/ΔNSm or Δ/Δ virus) showed efficacy in rat and sheep models and had no apparent adverse effects on fetal animals.[89,90] Other approaches have removed the NSm protein from the MP-12 virus (termed MP-12/ΔNSm).[91] The advantage of both of these recombinant deletion-based vaccines is the ability to differentiate infected from vaccinated animals based on differential detection of antigen-based immune responses by enzyme-linked immunosorbent assay.

Other vectored, replicon, and subunit vaccination strategies have been tested in laboratory animals.[92] A replication-defective chimpanzee adenovirus-based vaccine expressing the RVFV glycoproteins provides protection in experimentally infected sheep, goats, cattle, and camels[93] and is effective in a thermostabilized form, making it attractive for field use.[94] Many of these next-generation vaccine candidates could be used in both livestock and potentially humans; some are undergoing field testing to support veterinary approval,[95] but significant financial investment from endemic countries is needed to enable veterinary use. The most likely scenario is that, after a vaccine has demonstrated sufficient safety and efficacy in animals during outbreaks, the incentive may be there for testing and evaluation for human use in the event of a large-scale human outbreak.

PREVENTION OF ANIMAL AND HUMAN OUTBREAKS

The first step in the prevention of significant human disease is early detection of cases in animals through rigorous active surveillance and sentinel herd monitoring.[96] Once infected animals and/or herds are located, further spread can be prevented by mosquito control, animal movement control, ban on livestock slaughtering, or at least use of preventative measures (gloves, masks, and gowns) when handling carcasses or aborted fetuses. Public awareness and education as to the signs, symptoms, and risk factors are critical to prevent further animal disease and spread to people. Targeted vaccination of animals may be beneficial as a control measure in high-risk areas. Standard precautions prevent nosocomial transmission; risk to health care workers is low.[97]

POTENTIAL FOR EMERGENCE

RVFV has spread throughout Africa, to the island of Madagascar, and into the Saudi Arabian peninsula. Most recently, endemic RVF was discovered in both Angola and Nigeria.[98] Notably, human cases have not yet been recognized in these areas, potentially owing to focus on other diseases such as malaria, Yellow fever, and Dengue.

Concern over the further spread of RVF outside of Africa or the Saudi Arabian peninsula stems from the unexpected expansion of other arboviruses, namely West Nile, Chikungunya, and most recently Zika. Infected mosquitoes or livestock from Africa or the Middle East could introduce the virus into new locations via natural (migration) or mechanical (air travel, cargo) mechanisms. Importation of viremic livestock is believed to be responsible for spreading the virus into the Arabian peninsula.[99,100] Travel-associated cases of human RVF have occurred numerous times, most recently to China from Angola, and to France from both Mali and Zimbabwe,[101–103] without further transmission or establishment in the destination areas.

Although the risk of sporadic introduction of RVFV to the United States or Europe is likely high, the confluence of conditions necessary to allow sustained transmission and subsequent endemicity are probably rare.[104] North American mosquito species have the capacity to become infected with and potentially transmit RVFV.[105,106] The proximity of infected mosquito vectors and amplifying host animal populations, temperature, and rainfall conditions will all influence vector and virus survival, making accurate predictions of the likelihood of spread difficult.

Modeling studies are still unclear whether the virus would become enzootic in the United States if introduced via natural mechanisms.[107] By comparing the number of transmission days, livestock population, and proximity to potential entry points, the highest risk states include Texas, California, Nebraska, Minnesota, and New York.[6] Climate change may contribute to risk owing to increased environmental temperatures that extend mosquito survival time. California is at particular risk owing to a high density of both mosquitos and dairy cattle.[107]

Experiments have not yet been performed on whether or not resident North American wildlife, such as deer and elk, are capable of becoming hosts and contributing to enzootic maintenance. However, because many different mosquito species are competent for virus replication (see **Table 1**) and because a variety of wild animals in Africa are susceptible (see **Table 2**), it is conceivable that North American wild animals could also serve as hosts. RVFV replicates readily to high titers in cell lines from the white tailed deer,[108] although to date no experimental infections have been attempted in these animals.

Under the worst case scenario, the US Department of Agriculture believes the virus would become endemic within the United States in just 2 years, and would result in more than $50 billion in damages and control efforts.[104] Immediate costs during or after an outbreak in terms of human illness, loss of animals, disruption of animal supply chains, and mitigation efforts would be massive. Further losses economically include control policies and international trade restrictions imposed on US livestock to other countries.[5]

SUMMARY

RVF is a One Health disease that highlights the need to consider climate, veterinary health, and human behavior to prevent future outbreaks. Prevention of significant epizootics and epidemics is important in endemic areas owing to the severe economic impact. Also critical is prevention of spread to new areas.

REFERENCES

1. World Organization for Animal Health (OIE). OIE-Listed diseases, infections and infestations in force in 2016. Available at: http://www.oie.int/en/animal-health-in-the-world/oie-listed-diseases-2016/. Accessed August 24, 2016.
2. Daubney R, Hudson JR. Enzootic hepatitis or Rift Valley fever: an undescribed virus disease of sheep, cattle, and man from east Africa. J Pathol Bacteriol 1931; 34:545–79.
3. Weaver SC, Reisen WK. Present and future arboviral threats. Antiviral Res 2009; 85(2):328–45.
4. Chevalier V, Pepin M, Plee L, et al. Rift Valley fever–a threat for Europe? Euro Surveill 2010;15(10):19506.
5. Hartley DM, Rinderknecht JL, Nipp TL, et al, National Center for Foreign Animal and Zoonotic Disease Defense Advisory Group on Rift Valley Fever. Potential effects of Rift Valley fever in the United States. Emerg Infect Dis 2011;17(8):e1.
6. Konrad SK, Miller SN. A temperature-limited assessment of the risk of Rift Valley fever transmission and establishment in the continental United States of America. Geospat Health 2012;6(2):161–70.
7. US Department of Agriculture. 7 CFR Part 331 and 9 CFR Part 121. Agricultural Bioterrorism Protection Act of 2002; possession, use, and transfer of biological agents and toxins; final rule. Fed Reg 2005;70:13241–92.
8. US Department of Health and Human Services. 42 CFR parts 72, 73 and 42 CFR part 1003. Posession, use, and transfer of Select agents and toxins; final rule. Fed Reg 2005;70(52):13294–325.
9. Workshop on Prioritization of Pathogens. Blueprint for R&D preparedness and response to public health emergencies due to highly infectious pathogens.

World Health Organization; 2015. Available at: http://www.who.int/csr/research-and-development/meeting-report-prioritization.pdf?ua=1. Accessed February 22, 2017.

10. Cohen J. Unfilled Vials: scientifically feasible vaccines against major diseases are stalled for lack of funds. Science 2016;351(6268):16–9.

11. Ferron F, Li Z, Danek EI, et al. The hexamer structure of Rift Valley fever virus nucleoprotein suggests a mechanism for its assembly into ribonucleoprotein complexes. PLoS Pathog 2011;7(5):e1002030.

12. Le May N, Gauliard N, Billecocq A, et al. The N terminus of Rift Valley fever virus nucleoprotein is essential for dimerization. J Virol 2005;79(18):11974–80.

13. Anderson GW Jr, Smith JF. Immunoelectron microscopy of Rift Valley fever viral morphogenesis in primary rat hepatocytes. Virology 1987;161(1):91–100.

14. Bird BH, Githinji JW, Macharia JM, et al. Multiple virus lineages sharing recent common ancestry were associated with a Large Rift Valley fever outbreak among livestock in Kenya during 2006-2007. J Virol 2008;82(22):11152–66.

15. Bird BH, Khristova ML, Rollin PE, et al. Complete genome analysis of 33 ecologically and biologically diverse Rift Valley fever virus strains reveals widespread virus movement and low genetic diversity due to recent common ancestry. J Virol 2007;81(6):2805–16.

16. Sall AA, Zanotto PM, Sene OK, et al. Genetic reassortment of Rift Valley fever virus in nature. J Virol 1999;73(10):8196–200.

17. Linthicum KJ, Britch SC, Anyamba A. Rift Valley fever: an emerging mosquito-borne disease. Annu Rev Entomol 2016;61:395–415.

18. Clements AN. Arboviruses: case studies of transmission: Rift Valley fever virus. In: Clements AN, editor. Biology of mosquitoes: transmission of viruses and interactions with bacteria, vol. 3. Wallingford (Oxfordshire): GBR: CABI Publishing; 2012. p. 298.

19. Fontenille D, Traore-Lamizana M, Diallo M, et al. New vectors of Rift Valley fever in West Africa. Emerg Infect Dis 1998;4(2):289–93.

20. Davies FG, Highton RB. Possible vectors of Rift Valley fever in Kenya. Trans R Soc Trop Med Hyg 1980;74(6):815–6.

21. van Velden DJ, Meyer JD, Olivier J, et al. Rift Valley fever affecting humans in South Africa: a clinicopathological study. S Afr Med J 1977;51(24):867–71.

22. Linthicum KJ, Davies FG, Kairo A, et al. Rift Valley fever virus (family Bunyaviridae, genus Phlebovirus). Isolations from Diptera collected during an interepizootic period in Kenya. J Hyg (Lond) 1985;95(1):197–209.

23. Davies FG, Linthicum KJ, James AD. Rainfall and epizootic Rift Valley fever. Bull World Health Organ 1985;63(5):941–3.

24. Boiro I, Konstaninov OK, Numerov AD. Isolation of Rift Valley fever virus from bats in the Republic of Guinea. Bull Soc Pathol Exot Filiales 1987;80(1):62–7 [in French].

25. Capobianco Dondona A, Aschenborn O, Pinoni C, et al. Rift Valley fever virus among wild ruminants, Etosha National Park, Namibia, 2011. Emerg Infect Dis 2016;22(1):128–30.

26. Davies FG, Koros J, Mbugua H. Rift Valley fever in Kenya: the presence of antibody to the virus in camels (Camelus dromedarius). J Hyg (Lond) 1985;94(2):241–4.

27. McIntosh BM. Rift Valley fever. 1. Vector studies in the field. J S Afr Vet Med Assoc 1972;43(4):391–5.

28. LaBeaud AD, Pfeil S, Muiruri S, et al. Factors associated with severe human Rift Valley fever in Sangailu, Garissa County, Kenya. PLoS Negl Trop Dis 2015;9(3): e0003548.
29. Anyangu AS, Gould LH, Sharif SK, et al. Risk factors for severe Rift Valley fever infection in Kenya, 2007. Am J Trop Med Hyg 2010;83(2 Suppl):14–21.
30. Madani TA, Al-Mazrou YY, Al-Jeffri MH, et al. Rift Valley fever epidemic in Saudi Arabia: epidemiological, clinical, and laboratory characteristics. Clin Infect Dis 2003;37(8):1084–92.
31. Gear J, De Meillon B, Measroch V, et al. Rift Valley fever in South Africa. 2. The occurrence of human cases in the Orange Free State, the North-Western Cape Province, the Western and Southern Transvaal. B. Field and laboratory investigation. S Afr Med J 1951;25(49):908–12.
32. McIntosh BM, Russell D, dos Santos I, et al. Rift Valley fever in humans in South Africa. S Afr Med J 1980;58(20):803–6.
33. Dar O, McIntyre S, Hogarth S, et al. Rift Valley fever and a new paradigm of research and development for zoonotic disease control. Emerg Infect Dis 2013;19(2):189–93.
34. ProMed-mail. Rift Valley fever - Uganda (Kabale). 2016. 20160313.4090478. Available at: http://www.promedmail.org. Accessed September 2, 2016.
35. Lam Ayebe A. Uganda: Govt Confirms Rift Valley Fever Outbreak. 2016. Available at: http://allafrica.com/stories/201603220149.html. Accessed August 24, 2016.
36. Niklasson B, Liljestrand J, Bergstrom S, et al. Rift Valley fever: a sero-epidemiological survey among pregnant women in Mozambique. Epidemiol Infect 1987;99(2):517–22.
37. Adam I, Karsany MS. Case report: Rift Valley fever with vertical transmission in a pregnant Sudanese woman. J Med Virol 2008;80(5):929.
38. Arishi HM, Aqeel AY, Al Hazmi MM. Vertical transmission of fatal Rift Valley fever in a newborn. Ann Trop Paediatr 2006;26(3):251–3.
39. Smithburn KC, Mahaffy AF, Haddow AJ, et al. Rift Valley fever; accidental infections among laboratory workers. J Immunol 1949;62(2):213–27.
40. Francis T, Magill TP. Rift Valley fever: a report of three cases of laboratory infection and the experimental transmission of the disease to ferrets. J Exp Med 1935;62(3):433–48.
41. Kitchen SF. Laboratory infections with the virus of Rift Valley fever. Am J Trop Med 1934;14:547–64.
42. Schwentker FF, Rivers TM. Rift Valley fever in man: report of a fatal laboratory infection complicated by thrombophlebitis. J Exp Med 1934;59(3):305–13.
43. Sabin AB, Blumberg RW. Human infection with Rift Valley fever virus and immunity twelve years after single attack. Proc Soc Exp Biol Med 1947;64(4):385–9.
44. James Martin Center for Nonproliferation Studies. Chemical and biological weapons: possession and programs past and present. 2008. Available at: http://cns.miis.edu/cbw/possess.htm. Accessed July 9, 2015.
45. Leitenberg M, Zilinskas RA. The soviet biological weapons program: a history. Cambridge (MA): Harvard University Press; 2012.
46. Ellis J, Moon C. The US Biological Weapons Program. In: Wheelis M, Rozsa L, Dando M, editors. Deadly cultures: biological weapons since 1945. Cambridge (MA): Harvard University Press; 2006. p. 9–46.
47. Avery D. The Canadian Biological Weapons Program and the tripartite alliance. In: Wheelis M, Rozsa L, Dando M, editors. Deadly cultures: biological weapons since 1945. Cambridge (MA): Harvard University Press; 2006. p. 84–107.

48. International Institute for Peace and Conflict Research. The problem of chemical and biological warfare: volume I: the rise of CB weapons, vol. 1. Stockholm (Sweden): Almqvist & Wiksell; 1971.

49. Harris SH. Factories of death: Japanese biological warfare, 1932-45, and the American cover-up. New York: Routledge; 1994.

50. Bryden J. Deadly allies: Canada's secret war 1937-1947. Toronto (Canada): McClelland & Stewart, Inc.; 1989.

51. Millet P. Antianimal biological weapons programs. In: Wheelis M, Rozsa L, Dando M, editors. Deadly cultures: biological weapons since 1945. Cambridge (MA): Harvard University Press; 2006. p. 224–35.

52. Endicott S, Hagerman E. The United States and Biological Warfare: secrets from the early cold war and Korea. Indianapolis (IN): Indiana University Press; 1998.

53. Jones K. A brief history of the U.S. Army Project Fort Detrick Operation White-coat. Available at: http://usarmywhitecoat.com/?page_id=7. Accessed August 24, 2016.

54. Anderson AO. Infectious Disease and the Ethics of Human Volunteers in respect to the Whitecoat Project. Available at: http://usarmywhitecoat.com/wp-content/uploads/2013/12/1954-73-Op-Whitecoat-ID-Res-No-Video-press.pdf. Accessed August 25, 2015.

55. Mandell RB, Flick R. Rift Valley fever virus: a real bioterror threat. Bioterror Biodefense. 2011;2(2):108.

56. US Department of Health and Human Services. Biosafety in microbiological and biomedical laboratories. 5th edition. Washington, DC: U.S. Government Printing Office; 2009.

57. Coetzer JA. The pathology of Rift Valley fever. II. Lesions occurring in field cases in adult cattle, calves and aborted foetuses. Onderstepoort J Vet Res 1982; 49(1):11–7.

58. Coetzer JA. The pathology of Rift Valley fever. I. Lesions occurring in natural cases in new-born lambs. Onderstepoort J Vet Res 1977;44(4):205–11.

59. Van der Lugt JJ, Coetzer JA, Smit MM. Distribution of viral antigen in tissues of new-born lambs infected with Rift Valley fever virus. Onderstepoort J Vet Res 1996;63(4):341–7.

60. Laughlin LW, Meegan JM, Strausbaugh LJ, et al. Epidemic Rift Valley fever in Egypt: observations of the spectrum of human illness. Trans R Soc Trop Med Hyg 1979;73(6):630–3.

61. Freed I. Rift valley fever in man, complicated by retinal changes and loss of vision. S Afr Med J 1951;25(50):930–2.

62. Al-Hazmi A, Al-Rajhi AA, Abboud EB, et al. Ocular complications of Rift Valley fever outbreak in Saudi Arabia. Ophthalmology 2005;112(2):313–8.

63. Arthur RR, el-Sharkawy MS, Cope SE, et al. Recurrence of Rift Valley fever in Egypt. Lancet 1993;342(8880):1149–50.

64. Siam AL, Meegan JM, Gharbawi KF. Rift Valley fever ocular manifestations: observations during the 1977 epidemic in Egypt. Br J Ophthalmol 1980;64(5): 366–74.

65. Abdel-Wahab KS, El Baz LM, El-Tayeb EM, et al. Rift Valley fever virus infections in Egypt: pathological and virological findings in man. Trans R Soc Trop Med Hyg 1978;72(4):392–6.

66. Hise AG, Traylor Z, Hall NB, et al. Association of symptoms and severity of rift valley fever with genetic polymorphisms in human innate immune pathways. PLoS Negl Trop Dis 2015;9(3):e0003584.

67. Mohamed M, Mosha F, Mghamba J, et al. Epidemiologic and clinical aspects of a Rift Valley fever outbreak in humans in Tanzania, 2007. Am J Trop Med Hyg 2010;83(2 Suppl):22–7.

68. Haneche F, Leparc-Goffart I, Simon F, et al. Rift Valley fever in kidney transplant recipient returning from Mali with viral RNA detected in semen up to four months from symptom onset, France, autumn 2015. Euro Surveill 2016;21(18):2–5.

69. World Organization for Animal Health (OIE). List of Reference Experts and Laboratories. Available at: http://www.oie.int/en/our-scientific-expertise/reference-laboratories/list-of-laboratories/. Accessed September 19, 2016.

70. Huggins JW. Prospects for treatment of viral hemorrhagic fevers with ribavirin, a broad-spectrum antiviral drug. Rev Infect Dis 1989;11(S4):S750–61.

71. McCormick JB, King IJ, Webb PA, et al. Lassa fever. Effective therapy with ribavirin. N Engl J Med 1986;314(1):20–6.

72. van Eeden PJ, van Eeden SF, Joubert JR, et al. A nosocomial outbreak of Crimean-Congo haemorrhagic fever at Tygerberg Hospital. Part II. Management of patients. S Afr Med J 1985;68(10):718–21.

73. Bird BH, Reynes JM, Nichol ST. Rift Valley fever. In: Magill AJ, Strickland GT, Maguire JH, et al, editors. Hunter's tropical medicine and emerging infectious disease. 9th edition. Amsterdam: Elsevier Health Sciences; 2012. p. 340–3.

74. Caroline AL, Powell DS, Bethel LM, et al. Broad spectrum antiviral activity of favipiravir (T-705): protection from highly lethal inhalational Rift Valley Fever. PLoS Negl Trop Dis 2014;8(4):e2790.

75. Bird BH, Nichol ST. Breaking the chain: Rift Valley fever virus control via livestock vaccination. Curr Opin Virol 2012;2(3):315–23.

76. Committee on Special Immunizations Program for Laboratory Personnel Engaged in Research on Countermeasures for Select Agents. Protecting the frontline in biodefense research: the special immunizations program. Washington, DC: National Academies Press; 2011.

77. Randall R, Binn LN, Harrison VR. Immunization against Rift Valley fever virus. Studies on the immunogenicity of lyophilized formalin-inactivated vaccine. J Immunol 1964;93:293–9.

78. Kark JD, Aynor Y, Peters CJ. A Rift Valley fever vaccine trial. I. Side effects and serologic response over a six-month follow-up. Am J Epidemiol 1982;116(5):808–20.

79. Rusnak JM, Gibbs P, Boudreau E, et al. Immunogenicity and safety of an inactivated Rift Valley fever vaccine in a 19-year study. Vaccine 2011;29(17):3222–9.

80. Morrill JC, Jennings GB, Caplen H, et al. Pathogenicity and immunogenicity of a mutagen-attenuated Rift Valley fever virus immunogen in pregnant ewes. Am J Vet Res 1987;48(7):1042–7.

81. Makoschey B, van Kilsdonk E, Hubers WR, et al. Rift Valley fever vaccine virus clone 13 is able to cross the ovine placental barrier associated with foetal infections, malformations, and stillbirths. PLoS Negl Trop Dis 2016;10(3):e0004550.

82. Morrill JC, Mebus CA, Peters CJ. Safety of a mutagen-attenuated Rift Valley fever virus vaccine in fetal and neonatal bovids. Am J Vet Res 1997;58(10):1110–4.

83. Morrill JC, Mebus CA, Peters CJ. Safety and efficacy of a mutagen-attenuated Rift Valley fever virus vaccine in cattle. Am J Vet Res 1997;58(10):1104–9.

84. Morrill JC, Laughlin RC, Lokugamage N, et al. Safety and immunogenicity of recombinant Rift Valley fever MP-12 vaccine candidates in sheep. Vaccine 2013;31(3):559–65.

85. Ahmed Kamal S. Observations on rift valley fever virus and vaccines in Egypt. Virol J 2011;8:532.
86. Pittman PR, McClain D, Quinn X, et al. Safety and immunogenicity of a mutagenized, live attenuated Rift Valley fever vaccine, MP-12, in a Phase 1 dose escalation and route comparison study in humans. Vaccine 2016;34(4):424–9.
87. Pittman PR, Norris SL, Brown ES, et al. Rift Valley fever MP-12 vaccine phase 2 clinical trial: safety, immunogenicity, and genetic characterization of virus isolates. Vaccine 2016;34(4):523–30.
88. Pittman PR, Liu CT, Cannon TL, et al. Immunogenicity of an inactivated Rift Valley fever vaccine in humans: a 12-year experience. Vaccine 1999;18(1–2):181–9.
89. Bird BH, Albarino CG, Hartman AL, et al. Rift valley fever virus lacking the NSs and NSm genes is highly attenuated, confers protective immunity from virulent virus challenge, and allows for differential identification of infected and vaccinated animals. J Virol 2008;82(6):2681–91.
90. Bird BH, Maartens LH, Campbell S, et al. Rift Valley fever virus vaccine lacking the NSs and NSm genes is safe, nonteratogenic, and confers protection from viremia, pyrexia, and abortion following challenge in adult and pregnant sheep. J Virol 2011;85(24):12901–9.
91. Morrill JC, Laughlin RC, Lokugamage N, et al. Immunogenicity of a recombinant Rift Valley fever MP-12-NSm deletion vaccine candidate in calves. Vaccine 2013;31(43):4988–94.
92. Kortekaas J. One health approach to Rift Valley fever vaccine development. Antiviral Res 2014;106:24–32.
93. Warimwe GM, Gesharisha J, Carr BV, et al. Chimpanzee adenovirus vaccine provides multispecies protection against Rift Valley fever. Sci Rep 2016;6:20617.
94. Dulal P, Wright D, Ashfield R, et al. Potency of a thermostabilised chimpanzee adenovirus Rift Valley Fever vaccine in cattle. Vaccine 2016;34(20):2296–8.
95. Njenga MK, Njagi L, Thumbi SM, et al. Randomized controlled field trial to assess the immunogenicity and safety of Rift Valley fever clone 13 vaccine in livestock. PLoS Negl Trop Dis 2015;9(3):e0003550.
96. Davies FG, Martin V. Recognizing Rift Valley fever. Vet Ital 2006;42(1):31–53.
97. Al-Hamdan NA, Panackal AA, Al Bassam TH, et al. The risk of nosocomial transmission of Rift Valley fever. PLoS Negl Trop Dis 2015;9(12):e0004314.
98. ProMed-mail. Rift Valley fever - China (02): ex Angola, comment. 2016. 20160727.4371805. Available at: http://www.promedmail.org. Accessed September 2, 2016.
99. Abdo-Salem S, Waret-Szkuta A, Roger F, et al. Risk assessment of the introduction of Rift Valley fever from the Horn of Africa to Yemen via legal trade of small ruminants. Trop Anim Health Prod 2011;43(2):471–80.
100. Shoemaker T, Boulianne C, Vincent MJ, et al. Genetic analysis of viruses associated with emergence of Rift Valley fever in Saudi Arabia and Yemen, 2000-01. Emerg Infect Dis 2002;8(12):1415–20.
101. ProMed-mail. Rift Valley fever - China: ex Angola. 2016. 20160725.4368585. Available at: http://www.promedmail.org. Accessed September 2, 2016.
102. ProMed-mail. Rift Valley fever, human - France: ex Zimbabwe (Mashonaland East) first report. 2011. 20111020.3132. Available at: http://www.promedmail.org. Accessed September 2, 2016.
103. ProMed-mail. Rift Valley fever - France ex Mali, 2015. 2016. 20160506.4207036. Available at: http://www.promedmail.org. Accessed September 2, 2016.

104. Rolin AI, Berrang-Ford L, Kulkarni MA. The risk of Rift Valley fever virus introduction and establishment in the United States and European Union. Emerg Microbes Infect 2013;2(12):e81.
105. Turell MJ, Britch SC, Aldridge RL, et al. Potential for mosquitoes (Diptera: Culicidae) from Florida to transmit Rift valley fever virus. J Med Entomol 2013;50(5):1111–7.
106. Turell MJ, Byrd BD, Harrison BA. Potential for populations of Aedes J. Japonicus to transmit rift valley fever virus in the USA. J Am Mosq Control Assoc 2013;29(2):133–7.
107. Barker CM, Niu T, Reisen WK, et al. Data-driven modeling to assess receptivity for rift valley Fever virus. PLoS Negl Trop Dis 2013;7(11):e2515.
108. Gaudreault NN, Indran SV, Bryant PK, et al. Comparison of Rift Valley fever virus replication in North American livestock and wildlife cell lines. Front Microbiol 2015;6:664.
109. McIntosh BM, Dickinson DB, dos Santos I. Rift Valley fever. 3. Viraemia in cattle and sheep. 4. The susceptibility of mice and hamsters in relation to transmission of virus by mosquitoes. J S Afr Vet Assoc 1973;44(2):167–9.
110. Coetzer JA, Ishak KG. Sequential development of the liver lesions in new-born lambs infected with Rift Valley fever virus. I. Macroscopic and microscopic pathology. Onderstepoort J Vet Res 1982;49(2):103–8.
111. Coetzer JA, Ishak KG, Calvert RC. Sequential development of the liver lesions in new-born lambs infected with Rift Valley fever virus. II. Ultrastructural findings. Onderstepoort J Vet Res 1982;49(2):109–22.
112. Food and Agriculture Organization of the United Nations. Emergency preparedness planning: Rift Valley fever. Available at: http://www.fao.org/ag/againfo/resources/documents/AH/RVF198.htm. Accessed August 24, 2016.

Carbapenem-Resistant *Enterobacteriaceae*

Alina Iovleva, MD[a], Yohei Doi, MD, PhD[b],*

KEYWORDS

- Carbapenemase • KPC • Rapid diagnosis

KEY POINTS

- Carbapenem-resistant *Enterobacteriaceae* (CRE) have spread in health care settings worldwide in the last decade.
- Timely and accurate detection of CRE, in particular those producing carbapenemase is of paramount importance to guide clinicians and inform infection preventionists.
- Several phenotypic and genotypic methods are available for rapid detection of carbapenemase production that can be implemented and performed in clinical microbiology laboratories.
- Treatment usually consists of combination of active antimicrobial agents, but newer agents with improved activity and safety profiles are in late-stage clinical development.

INTRODUCTION

Carbapenem antibiotics are generally considered to be the most potent group of antimicrobial agents with proven efficacy in the treatment of patients with severe bacterial infections, including those caused by otherwise antimicrobial-resistant strains. The recent increase in the rates of carbapenem-resistant *Enterobacteriaceae* (CRE) among health care-associated *Enterobacteriaceae* species, in particular *Klebsiella pneumoniae*, is therefore a major cause for concern. This surge in CRE is mostly driven by the emergence and spread of carbapenemases, a specific group of β-lactamases that are capable of hydrolyzing carbapenems. Most strains that produce carbapenemases are resistant to carbapenems, and those that are not demonstrate reduced susceptibility to these agents.

Funding: The effort of Y. Doi was supported by research grants from the National Institutes of Health (R01AI104895, R21AI123747).
Transparency Declarations: Y. Doi has served on advisory boards for Meiji, Achaogen, Allergan, Curetis, and has received research funding from The Medicines Company for a study unrelated to this work. A. Iovleva declares no conflicts of interest.
[a] Division of Infectious Diseases, University of Pittsburgh School of Medicine, Falk Medical Building, Suite 3A, 3601 Fifth Avenue, Pittsburgh, PA 15213, USA; [b] Division of Infectious Diseases, University of Pittsburgh School of Medicine, S829 Scaife Hall, 3550 Terrace Street, Pittsburgh, PA 15261, USA
* Corresponding author.
E-mail address: yod4@pitt.edu

Clin Lab Med 37 (2017) 303–315
http://dx.doi.org/10.1016/j.cll.2017.01.005
0272-2712/17/© 2017 Elsevier Inc. All rights reserved.

labmed.theclinics.com

Three groups of carbapenemases—KPC, NDM, and OXA-48—are currently considered to be the 3 major β-lactamases of epidemiologic and clinical significance. In the United States, KPC is by far the most common carbapenemase produced by CRE,[1] but outbreaks of NDM-producing *Enterobacteriaceae* have been reported from US hospitals[2,3]; OXA-48–producing *Enterobacteriaceae* strains have also been reported sporadically.[4] It is essential that clinical microbiology laboratories be capable of recognizing CRE strains that produce these key groups of carbapenemases and refer them for further testing when appropriate to inform clinicians and infection preventionists. This review is intended to provide clinical microbiologists with an overview of the epidemiology, diagnosis, and clinical implications of CRE.

HISTORY OF CARBAPENEM-RESISTANT *ENTEROBACTERIACEAE*

The discovery and clinical application of antimicrobial agents constitutes one of the greatest public health achievements of the 20th century, drastically reducing mortality from common infectious diseases like pneumonia and diarrheal illnesses.[5] However, the introduction of every new class of antimicrobial agents has been eclipsed by the emergence of bacteria that are resistant to them. β-Lactams, arguably the most successful antimicrobial class used in clinical practice, have not been an exception in this regard. The introduction of ampicillin as an anti–Gram-negative aminopenicillin in the 1960s was quickly followed by the spread of *Escherichia coli* that produce TEM-1 β-lactamase, which is capable of hydrolyzing ampicillin.[6] To counter this, various oxyimino-cephalosporins (eg, cefotaxime, ceftazidime) were introduced in the 1980s, which were by design stable against hydrolysis by TEM-1 or SHV-1 (β-lactamase naturally produced by K pneumoniae and conferring ampicillin resistance). However, *Enterobacteriaceae* countered them several years later by generating variants of TEM-1 and SHV-1, which have extended the spectrum of hydrolysis to include not only aminopenicillins but also oxyimino-cephalosporins (thus the name extended-spectrum β-lactamases [ESBLs]).[6] ESBL producers were resistant to oxyimino-cephalosporins. Carbapenems were then introduced to clinics in the late 1980s and proved highly efficacious in the treatment of ESBL-producing K pneumoniae infections.[7]

Unfortunately, even carbapenems were not immune to the remarkable ability of *Enterobacteriaceae* to adapt to selective pressure. In the early 1990s, CRE emerged in Japan, followed by neighboring countries.[8] These strains produced metallo-β-lactamase (MBL) IMP-1, which was capable of hydrolyzing carbapenems and was encoded on plasmids that could transfer from one species to another. This was followed by discovery of VIM-1, another acquired MBL, which was initially identified from *Pseudomonas aeruginosa* in Italy and subsequently found in *Enterobacteriaceae*.[9] In the United States, a K pneumoniae strain with resistance to carbapenems was identified in 1996. This strain produced a novel carbapenemase that was later coined KPC for K pneumoniae carbapenemase.[10] This KPC gene is encoded on a transferable plasmid and the enzyme is capable of hydrolyzing both oxyimino-cephalosporins and carbapenems efficiently. It became apparent by the early 2000s that KPC-producing K pneumoniae was rapidly becoming endemic at hospitals in parts of New York City.[11,12] Since then, KPC-producing K pneumoniae has spread across the continental United States and many other countries worldwide causing both outbreaks and endemicity in certain regions.[1]

In parallel to the expansion of KPC in the United States and elsewhere, another group of carbapenemases, OXA-48, emerged and spread mostly in K pneumoniae in the Mediterranean countries in the 2000s.[13,14] More recently, a novel group of MBL, NDM (New Delhi metallo-β-lactamase), was identified and reported in carbapenem-resistant *K pneumoniae* and *E coli* in a patient who had traveled from India in 2009.[15] NDM-1 has since spread explosively in South Asia and also globally.[16,17]

CARBAPENEM-RESISTANT *ENTEROBACTERIACEAE* AND CARBAPENEMASE-PRODUCING *ENTEROBACTERIACEAE*

Both the terms CRE and CPE (carbapenemase-producing *Enterobacteriaceae*) appear in the literature and are sometimes used interchangeably. Although there is certainly a significant overlap between CRE and CPE, it is important to distinguish them because the former refers to the resistance phenotype, whereas the latter is defined by the mechanism underlying the phenotype. Carbapenemase production is certainly the most prominent mechanism underlying carbapenem resistance in Gram-negative pathogens. Other mechanisms such as overproduction of AmpC or production of ESBL can function together with outer membrane protein deficiency and overproduction of certain efflux pumps to confer carbapenem resistance, especially in species such as *Enterobacter* spp. In contrast, carbapenemase production usually results in clinically relevant levels of carbapenem resistance, but on occasion may only yield reduced susceptibility that does not reach the susceptibility breakpoints. Although CRE poses challenges with treatment in general, CPE is considered to be a more significant concern for both infection prevention and treatment because carbapenemase genes are carried mostly on plasmids that have the ability to transfer between bacterial species. Consequently, outbreaks owing to CPE are reported commonly, and CPE infections are associated with high mortality.[12,18] Rapid detection of CPE facilitates timely implementation of appropriate infection prevention measures, in addition to informing clinicians, who must decide on treatment regimens for CRE and CPE infections.

SPECTRUM OF RESISTANCE CONFERRED BY CARBAPENEMASES

The 3 major groups of carbapenemases belong to separate molecular classes as defined by Ambler[19]: KPC belongs to class A, NDM to class B, and OXA-48 to class D (**Table 1**). KPC uses a serine residue for its activity and has a very broad spectrum of substrates, including penicillins, cephalosporins, classic β-lactamase inhibitors (clavulanic acid, sulbactam and tazobactam), aztreonam, and carbapenems. Its activity is inhibited only minimally by clavulanic acid, but is inhibited well by boronic acid compounds.[20] MBLs including NDM are metalloenzymes that possess zinc in the active site. The spectrum of hydrolysis is similar to that of KPC, but spares aztreonam. Therefore, resistance to carbapenems and susceptibility to aztreonam is suggestive of MBL production; however, coproduction of ESBL is common in clinical strains, which make them also resistant to aztreonam.[21] OXA-48 is a serine β-lactamase like KPC, but has a unique spectrum of activity that includes penicillins and carbapenems yet spares cephalosporins and aztreonam. In addition, its activity against carbapenems is not as robust as that of KPC and MBLs. For this reason, detection of OXA-48-producing *Enterobacteriaceae* based on susceptibility phenotype is more challenging and requires attention to subtle irregularities, such as reduced susceptibility to carbapenems (eg, ertapenem minimum inhibitory concentration of ≥0.5 mg/L, or imipenem or meropenem minimum inhibitory concentration of ≥1 mg/L), which may not meet the current criteria for intermediate resistance or resistance.[22]

EPIDEMIOLOGY OF CARBAPENEM-RESISTANT *ENTEROBACTERIACEAE*

The prevalence of CRE as well as the types of common carbapenemases is highly dependent on geography, but the highest rates are seen in *K pneumoniae* over other

Table 1
Characteristics of major acquired carbapenemases in *Enterobacteriaceae*

	KPC	NDM	OXA-48
Molecular class	A	B	D
Common species	*K pneumoniae*	*K pneumoniae* *E coli*	*K pneumoniae*
Regions/countries with high burden	United States Brazil Italy Greece Israel China	South Asia (India, Pakistan, Bangladesh, Nepal)	Mediterranean (Turkey, Algeria, Lebanon, Libya, Tunisia, Morocco) Gulf (Saudi Arabia)
Spectrum of resistance	All β-lactams including carbapenems	All β-lactams including carbapenems but except aztreonam	Penicillins and carbapenems
Inhibited by classic β-lactamase inhibitors	Minimally	No	No
Inhibited by avibactam	Yes	No	Yes

species of the family *Enterobacteriaceae* across regions. It is also seen almost exclusively in health care–associated infections, with the exception of the Indian subcontinent where community-associated CRE infections owing to NDM-producing strains have been reported.[23] Countries known to have high overall rates of CRE include Greece, Italy, Brazil, and China, followed by several other countries including the United States and Colombia. Countries in the Indian subcontinent have a high burden of CRE that is driven by the spread of NDM-producing strains, but prevalence data are scarce. CRE rates among *K pneumoniae* are as high as 62% in Greece and 33% in Italy.[24] In the United States, 11% of *K pneumoniae* causing health care–associated infections were resistant to carbapenems in 2014, representing a modest decrease from 2013 (13%).[25] The majority of CRE cases are concentrated in the mid-Atlantic (New York, New Jersey, and Pennsylvania), the Midwest (Michigan and Illinois), and the Southeast (Florida).[26]

Globally, KPC is the most commonly observed carbapenemase in *Enterobacteriaceae*, and KPC-2 and KPC-3 are by far the most predominant alleles.[1] Countries with an high prevalence of KPC-producing *K pneumoniae* include the United States, as well as some countries in South America (Brazil and Colombia), Europe (Italy and Greece), and East Asia (China in particular). Most CREs in the United States produce KPC carbapenemases.[27] KPC-producing *K pneumoniae* is characterized by its clonality, in that the majority of the strains circulating globally belong to clonal complex (CC) 258 as defined by multilocus sequence typing. This suggests that CC258 acquired the KPC gene at an early stage in this epidemic and spread successfully.[28] The most common sequence type (ST) is ST258 in the United States, but other CC258 STs such as ST11, ST340, ST437, and ST512 predominate in countries outside the United States.[29]

NDM is the most common carbapenemase in the Indian subcontinent (India, Pakistan, and Bangladesh), and also possibly in some of the Balkan nations.[30] Although many NDM variants have been reported, NDM-1 continues to be the most frequent allele in this group of carbapenemases. NDM-producing *Enterobacteriaceae* are also increasingly reported from China, but the overall epidemiology there is yet unclear because their prevalence is typically reported from single hospitals or locales.[31] Organisms producing NDM carbapenemases have been sporadic in the United States and are associated mostly with direct importation from the Indian subcontinent,[32] although some locally acquired cases may be emerging.[33] Unlike with KPC-producing *K pneumoniae*, where CC258 is the predominant clonal lineage, the spread of NDM-producing *Enterobacteriaceae* is better explained by horizontal transfer of epidemic broad host-range plasmids carrying the NDM gene.[34]

OXA-48 is the third globally distributed group of carbapenemases, which comprises the canonical OXA-48 as well as its variants OXA-181 and OXA-232.[34] Outbreak reports of OXA-48–producing *Enterobacteriaceae* are concentrated in European and Mediterranean countries including North Africa, whereas sporadic cases have been identified in the United States, often in association with recent travel to India.[4,22]

DETECTION OF CARBAPENEMASES

Several approaches have been developed to identify the presence of carbapenemases in *Enterobacteriaceae*. These include phenotypic and genotypic (nuclear amplification-based) tests. Below is a brief overview of currently available methods.

PHENOTYPIC TESTS
Modified Hodge Test

In the modified Hodge test (MHT), a tenth dilution of McFarland 0.5 suspension of *E coli* ATCC 25922, is used to inoculate a Mueller-Hinton agar plate evenly, and a 10-μg imipenem disk is placed in the center of the plate. The suspected CPE strain is then streaked from the edge of the disk to the periphery of the plate to form a straight line of thick inoculum. After overnight incubation, if a carbapenemase is produced by the test strain, imipenem in the agar plate is hydrolyzed, allowing the susceptible *E coli* in the background to grow in toward the disk, creating a cloverleaf-like appearance.[35] The sensitivity and specificity of the MHT was shown to be excellent in detecting KPC-producing strains earlier in the CRE epidemic, making it one of the recommended confirmation tests of CPE by the Clinical and Laboratory Standards Institute. However, the technique is somewhat operator dependent, and occasional false-positive results produced by AmpC-producing strains make interpretation difficult. In addition, the MHT lacks the desired sensitivity in detecting MBL-producing strains.[36] Nonetheless, the MHT does not require any special supplies and detects KPC producers well, and therefore can still be useful in settings where resources are limited and KPC is the predominant carbapenemase.

Carbapenem Inactivation Method

The carbapenem inactivation method is a more recently described test to detect CPE.[37] With the carbapenem inactivation method, a 10-μg meropenem disk is first incubated in a suspension of the test strain at 35°C for 2 hours. After incubation, the meropenem disk is removed from the solution and placed on a Mueller Hinton agar plate inoculated with susceptible *E coli* as with the MHT. If carbapenemase is produced, the meropenem in the disk would have been inactivated during the initial incubation, allowing for uninhibited growth of *E coli*, making it appear as if the susceptible *E coli* is resistant. If no carbapenemase is produced, a clear inhibition zone is formed. This method has been validated against *Enterobacteriaceae* strains producing KPC, OXA-48, NDM, VIM, and IMP carbapenemases, with sensitivity reaching

99%.[38] It is low cost and does not require any special supplies or skills. For these reasons, it is now endorsed as one of the first-line confirmation tests of CPE by the Clinical and Laboratory Standards Institute.

Ethylenediaminetetraacetic Acid Inhibition Test

The ability of ethylenediaminetetraacetic acid (EDTA) to chelate metal ions makes it a useful compound in detecting MBL, because the activity of these enzymes depends on zinc ions.[39] With the EDTA inhibition test, an EDTA solution is added to a carbapenem disk, which is then placed on a plate inoculated with the strain of interest. If MBL is present, a larger zone of inhibition will form around the EDTA–carbapenem disk compared with the carbapenem disk without EDTA (control).[40] The same principle can be applied to other metal chelators such as sodium mercaptoacetic acid.[41]

Boronic Acid Inhibition Test

Boronic acid compounds have been known to be excellent inhibitors of class C β-lactamases[42], used for the detection of this group of enzymes[43] but, more recently, recognized as an excellent inhibitor of class A carbapenemases, including KPC. This property has been applied in detecting production of KPC carbapenemase.[44] With this test, 300 or 400 µg of 2-aminophenyl boronic acid is applied to an ertapenem or meropenem disk. An increase in the zone of inhibition of 5 mm or greater compared with the ertapenem or meropenem disk alone (control) is indicative of KPC production.

CARBA NP TEST

The Carba NP Test, originally developed by the group led by Drs Patrice Nordmann and Laurent Poirel, is a rapid colorimetric test that is based on the detection of pH changes that accompany hydrolysis of imipenem by carbapenemases.[45] In the original Carba NP test, the test strain first undergoes a lysis step, then the lysate is added to a solution consisting of imipenem monohydrate, phenol red and $ZnSO_4$ (initial pH of 7.8). This final solution is then incubated at 37°C for up to 2 hours. If carbapenemase is produced, the imipenem is hydrolyzed, resulting in reduction of the pH and color change from red to orange or yellow (**Fig. 1**). Although 2 hours of incubation is recommended, KPC producers can be detected in as little as 10 minutes. The Carba NP test is highly sensitive in detecting KPC and most MBL-producing strains. However, it may have difficulty identifying activity of relatively weak carbapenemases such as OXA-48 and GES-5, and also some mucoid strains.[46] The Carba NP test is one of the methods endorsed by the Clinical and Laboratory Standards Institute for the detection of carbapenemase production.

Matrix-Assisted Laser Desorption/Ionization Time-of-Flight Mass Spectrometry

Matrix-assisted laser desorption/ionization time-of-flight mass spectrometry assays to detect carbapenemase activity have been developed by many investigators.[47] Instruments that are currently used in clinical microbiology laboratories, such as Bruker Microflex (Bruker, Billerica, MA), can be used for this purpose. Although the details vary, a colony of the test strain is suspended in a solution containing a carbapenem and incubated at 37°C for a period ranging from 15 minutes to as long as several hours. A small fraction of this solution is loaded onto a target plate with a matrix after which mass spectra are acquired. For example, imipenem has an m/z of 300, and its dominant metabolite has an m/z of 254. Therefore, predominant detection of the latter peak relative to that of the intact imipenem indicates production of carbapenemase. A

No imipenem   With imipenem

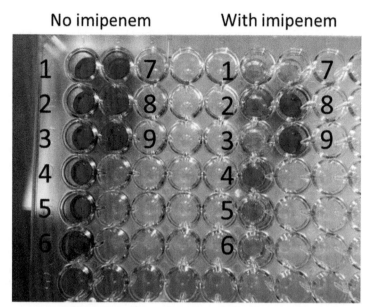

Fig. 1. Example of Carba NP test. Wells 1 to 7 are carbapenemase-producing strains, wells 8 and 9 are non–carbapenemase-producing strains. Photographed after 1 hour of reaction.

sensitivity and specificity of nearly100% has been reported, with a turnaround time as short as 30 minutes.[48,49] However, false-negative results with OXA-48–producing strains and slime-producing strains owing to interactions with polysaccharide have been reported. Although most published protocols use pure culture, successful use of bacteria collected directly from positive blood cultures have also been reported.[50] Although the protocol and analysis are yet to be standardized, the use of matrix-assisted laser desorption/ionisation time-of-flight mass spectrometry seems to be a practical option for laboratories that have access to this technology.

MOLECULAR TESTS
Conventional Polymerase Chain Reaction/Real-time Polymerase Chain Reaction

Detection of carbapenemase genes can be achieved by conventional or real-time polymerase chain reaction. Multiplex polymerase chain reaction assays for the common carbapenemase genes have been developed and can be used in settings where such assays are available.

Verigene

Verigene Gram-negative blood culture assay (Luminex Corporation, Austin, TX) is a nonamplified test that relies on nucleic acid extraction from positive blood cultures, followed by microarray-based detection using capture and detection probes. The test requires approximately 5 minutes of hands-on time and 2 hours to run. In addition to identification of 8 Gram-negative species, it is capable of detecting bla_{CTX-M}, bla_{KPC}, bla_{NDM}, bla_{VIM}, bla_{IMP}, and bla_{OXA} (including bla_{OXA-48}). The positive percentage agreement in the multicenter validation study was as follows: bla_{CTX-M}, 98.9%; bla_{KPC}, 100%; bla_{NDM}, 96.2%; bla_{OXA}, 94.3%; bla_{VIM}, 100%; and bla_{IMP}, 100%.[51] The materials cost is approximately $60 to $80 per test.[52]

BioFire FilmArray

The FilmArray Blood Culture Identification Panel (bioMérieux, Marcy-l'Étoile, France) is an automated multiplex polymerase chain reaction system that is carried out in a closed, disposable, single-use pouch.[53] It is primarily geared toward the rapid identification of bacteremia and fungemia directly from positive blood culture bottles, but it is also able to detect the presence of bla_{KPC} along with $mecA$ and $vanA/vanB$.[54] The hands-on time for sample preparation is 2 to 3 minutes, and the results are available in about 1 hour. A sensitivity and specificity of 100% has been reported for the detection of bla_{KPC}. However, a test on FilmArray costs more than $100, which limits the specific usefulness of this platform in detection bla_{KPC} in low to moderate prevalence settings. In addition, a negative test may not be informative in locales where other types of carbapenemases are found.

Xpert

The Xpert Carba-R (Cepheid, Sunnyvale, CA) detects bla_{KPC}, bla_{NDM}, bla_{VIM}, bla_{IMP}, and bla_{OXA-48}. The system has been approved for use in rectal swab specimens in the United States. The test requires a hands-on time of 1 minute and a run time of less than an hour, and can be run on an existing GeneXpert platform. The sensitivity, specificity, and positive and negative predictive values of the Xpert Carba-R assay compared with those of the reference culture and sequencing results have been reported to be 96.6%, 98.6%, 95.3%, and 99.0%, respectively.[55] Because the Xpert Carba-R only detects the presence of carbapenemase genes, information regarding the species carrying them (eg, $K pneumoniae$) is not available.

Genome and Metagenome Sequencing

Conceptually, whole-genome sequencing is an attractive method for the detection of carbapenemase genes because it can identify known as well as yet unknown genes that encode carbapenemases. An added advantage is that it will also yield information regarding species, clades, and any resistance genes other than carbapenemase genes. The cost of whole-genome sequencing has decreased precipitously over the last decade, to a point that application in clinical microbiology laboratories is in sight. However, there are several hurdles that need to be overcome before the technology can be incorporated into routine clinical microbiology, including turnaround time and data management.[56]

Metagenome sequencing uses similar technology as whole-genome sequencing, but instead of using pure culture DNA as the starting material, it uses DNA extracted directly from biological specimens such as sputum. Because of the high cost and complexity of the data analysis, it is currently evaluated for the diagnosis of infections for which currently available diagnostic methods do not suffice. This technique will be able to detect carbapenemase genes present in the specimens tested; however, it will not provide information on the species of the strain(s) producing carbapenemase.

TREATMENT OF CARBAPENEM-RESISTANT ENTEROBACTERIACEAE INFECTIONS
Currently Available Therapy

CRE strains are usually resistant to all β-lactam agents, including carbapenems and β-lactamase inhibitor combinations (with a notable exception of ceftazidime-avibactam). The majority of these strains are still susceptible to polymyxins (colistin and polymyxin B) and tigecycline. Additionally some KPC-producing and OXA-48–producing strains are susceptible to aminoglycosides (gentamicin or amikacin). NDM-producing strains are typically resistant to all aminoglycosides.

Because polymyxins and tigecycline do not have the most desirable pharmacokinetic properties, mortality of patients with invasive CRE infections is high when treated with a single active agent (monotherapy). Therefore, treatment with 2 or more active agents (combination therapy) is considered routinely.[57] There are no published, randomized, clinical trials that specifically address treatment of CRE infections at this time, and the best available data are retrospective cohort studies examining treatment and mortality outcome of patients with invasive CRE infections. In a systematic review of the clinical outcome of CRE infections in 889 patients, most of which were owing to KPC-producing *K pneumoniae*, 441 received combination therapy, 346 received monotherapy, and 102 received inactive therapy.[58] The mortality rates of monotherapy were 40.1% for carbapenem, 41.1% for tigecycline, and 42.8% for colistin, whereas the mortality for inactive therapy was 46.1%. In contrast, the mortality rates for combination therapy were 30.7% for carbapenem-sparing combinations and 18.8% for carbapenem-containing combinations. Based on these data, carbapenem-containing regimens (such as meropenem combined with colistin, tigecycline, or gentamicin) are frequently used for the treatment of invasive CRE infections. It has also been suggested that when the KPC-producing *K pneumoniae* develops resistance to colistin but remains susceptible to gentamicin, gentamicin-containing regimens may be associated with lower mortality.[59]

New Agents in Development

There are multiple new agents that are in clinical development and have activity against CRE. They can be divided into β-lactam/β-lactamase inhibitor combinations and others. Among them, ceftazidime-avibactam has been available for clinical use in the United States since 2015. Avibactam is a novel β-lactamase inhibitor that inhibits KPC, ESBL, AmpC, and OXA-48. As a result, the ceftazidime-avibactam combination is active against most KPC– and OXA-48–producing strains. However, it is not active against MBL-producing strains, including those producing NDM.[60] Although efficacy data are scarce, a 30-day mortality of 24% has been reported in a case series of CRE infections treated with ceftazidime-avibactam, which is reasonably low when considering the ill patient population.[61] However, resistance to ceftazidime-avibactam, either intrinsic or acquired, has already been reported. This raises the question whether this agent can be used as monotherapy or should be used in the context of combination therapy to prevent emergence of resistance.[33,61] Two other β-lactam/β-lactamase inhibitor combinations are in late-stage clinical development, including meropenem-vaborbactam and imipenem-cilastatin-relebactam. Although the structures of the inhibitors and the partner agents differ, the overall spectrum of activity of these agents is similar to that of ceftazidime-avibactam.[62] Agents from other classes in late-stage clinical development include plazomicin, eravacycline, and cefiderocol. Plazomicin is a new aminoglycoside derived from sisomicin and designed to resist most aminoglycoside-modifying enzymes. It is active against most *Enterobacteriaceae* strains, including KPC-producing strains, but activity against NDM-producing strains is limited owing to frequent coproduction of 16S ribosomal RNA methyltransferase, which confers resistance to aminoglycosides including plazomicin. Eravacycline is a novel fluorocycline of the tetracycline class with broad activity against Gram-negative bacteria including CRE. Its spectrum of activity is similar to that of tigecycline, but it may have an advantage in terms of in vitro activity, pharmacokinetics, and tolerability.[62] Finally, cefiderocol (S-649266) is a novel siderophore cephalosporin with a catechol moiety that demonstrates in vitro activity against CRE, including both KPC-producing and MBL-producing *Enterobacteriaceae*.[63] The availability of these new anti-CRE agents is expected to transform treatment approaches for invasive CRE infections in the very near future.

SUMMARY

CRE has spread in health care settings worldwide in the last decade. CRE infections are notoriously difficult to treat and associated with high mortality because of limited treatment options. Timely and accurate detection of CRE, in particular those producing carbapenemase, or CPE, is therefore of paramount importance both to guide clinicians and to inform infection preventionists. Several phenotypic and genetic methods are available for rapid detection of carbapenemase production, many of which, especially the phenotypic ones, can be implemented in regular clinical microbiology laboratories. Treatment of CRE infections usually consist of combination of active antimicrobial agents, but newer agents with improved activity and safety are in clinical development, some of which we expect to become available for clinical use in the near future.

REFERENCES

1. Munoz-Price LS, Poirel L, Bonomo RA, et al. Clinical epidemiology of the global expansion of *Klebsiella pneumoniae* carbapenemases. Lancet Infect Dis 2013; 13:785–96.
2. Epson EE, Pisney LM, Wendt JM, et al. Carbapenem-resistant *Klebsiella pneumoniae* producing New Delhi metallo-β-lactamase at an acute care hospital, Colorado, 2012. Infect Control Hosp Epidemiol 2014;35:390–7.
3. Epstein L, Hunter JC, Arwady MA, et al. New Delhi metallo-β-lactamase-producing carbapenem-resistant *Escherichia coli* associated with exposure to duodenoscopes. JAMA 2014;312:1447–55.
4. Lyman M, Walters M, Lonsway D, et al. Notes from the field: carbapenem-resistant Enterobacteriaceae producing OXA-48-like carbapenemases–United States, 2010-2015. MMWR Morb Mortal Wkly Rep 2015;64:1315–6.
5. Centers for Disease Control and Prevention. Ten great public health achievements–United States, 1900-1999. MMWR Morb Mortal Wkly Rep 1999;48:241–3.
6. Paterson DL, Bonomo RA. Extended-spectrum β-lactamases: a clinical update. Clin Microbiol Rev 2005;18:657–86.
7. Paterson DL, Ko WC, Von Gottberg A, et al. Antibiotic therapy for *Klebsiella pneumoniae* bacteremia: implications of production of extended-spectrum β-lactamases. Clin Infect Dis 2004;39:31–7.
8. Osano E, Arakawa Y, Wacharotayankun R, et al. Molecular characterization of an enterobacterial metallo β-lactamase found in a clinical isolate of *Serratia marcescens* that shows imipenem resistance. Antimicrob Agents Chemother 1994;38: 71–8.
9. Lauretti L, Riccio ML, Mazzariol A, et al. Cloning and characterization of bla_{VIM}, a new integron-borne metallo-β-lactamase gene from a *Pseudomonas aeruginosa* clinical isolate. Antimicrob Agents Chemother 1999;43:1584–90.
10. Yigit H, Queenan AM, Anderson GJ, et al. Novel carbapenem-hydrolyzing β-lactamase, KPC-1, from a carbapenem-resistant strain of *Klebsiella pneumoniae*. Antimicrob Agents Chemother 2001;45:1151–61.
11. Bradford PA, Bratu S, Urban C, et al. Emergence of carbapenem-resistant *Klebsiella* species possessing the class A carbapenem-hydrolyzing KPC-2 and inhibitor-resistant TEM-30 β-lactamases in New York City. Clin Infect Dis 2004; 39:55–60.
12. Bratu S, Landman D, Haag R, et al. Rapid spread of carbapenem-resistant *Klebsiella pneumoniae* in New York City: a new threat to our antibiotic armamentarium. Arch Intern Med 2005;165:1430–5.

13. Poirel L, Heritier C, Tolun V, et al. Emergence of oxacillinase-mediated resistance to imipenem in *Klebsiella pneumoniae*. Antimicrob Agents Chemother 2004;48: 15–22.

14. Potron A, Poirel L, Rondinaud E, et al. Intercontinental spread of OXA-48 β-lactamase-producing Enterobacteriaceae over a 11-year period, 2001 to 2011. Euro Surveill 2013;18 [pii: 20549].

15. Yong D, Toleman MA, Giske CG, et al. Characterization of a new metallo-β-lactamase gene, bla_{NDM-1}, and a novel erythromycin esterase gene carried on a unique genetic structure in *Klebsiella pneumoniae* sequence type 14 from India. Antimicrob Agents Chemother 2009;53:5046–54.

16. Kumarasamy KK, Toleman MA, Walsh TR, et al. Emergence of a new antibiotic resistance mechanism in India, Pakistan, and the UK: a molecular, biological, and epidemiological study. Lancet Infect Dis 2010;10:597–602.

17. Nordmann P, Poirel L, Walsh TR, et al. The emerging NDM carbapenemases. Trends Microbiol 2011;19:588–95.

18. Tumbarello M, Viale P, Viscoli C, et al. Predictors of mortality in bloodstream infections caused by *Klebsiella pneumoniae* carbapenemase-producing *K. pneumoniae*: importance of combination therapy. Clin Infect Dis 2012;55:943–50.

19. Ambler RP. The structure of β-lactamases. Philos Trans R Soc Lond B Biol Sci 1980;289:321–31.

20. Ke W, Bethel CR, Papp-Wallace KM, et al. Crystal structures of KPC-2 β-lactamase in complex with 3-nitrophenyl boronic acid and the penam sulfone PSR-3-226. Antimicrob Agents Chemother 2012;56:2713–8.

21. Bonomo RA. New Delhi metallo-β-lactamase and multidrug resistance: a global SOS? Clin Infect Dis 2011;52:485–7.

22. Poirel L, Potron A, Nordmann P. OXA-48-like carbapenemases: the phantom menace. J Antimicrob Chemother 2012;67:1597–606.

23. Borah VV, Saikia KK, Chandra P, et al. New Delhi metallo-β-lactamase and extended spectrum β-lactamases co-producing isolates are high in community-acquired urinary infections in Assam as detected by a novel multiplex polymerase chain reaction assay. Indian J Med Microbiol 2016;34:173–82.

24. European Centre for Disease Prevention and Control. Antimicrobial resistance surveillance in Europe, 2014. 2015. Available at: http://ecdc.europa.eu/en/publications/Publications/antimicrobial-resistance-europe-2014.pdf. Accessed November 27, 2016.

25. Weiner LM, Webb AK, Limbago B, et al. Antimicrobial-resistant pathogens associated with healthcare-associated infections: summary of data reported to the National Healthcare Safety Network at the Centers for Disease Control and Prevention, 2011-2014. Infect Control Hosp Epidemiol 2016;37:1288–301.

26. The Center for Disease Dynamics Economics and Policy. Resistance Map. 2016. Available at: http://resistancemap.cddep.org/. Accessed November 27, 2016.

27. Castanheira M, Farrell SE, Krause KM, et al. Contemporary diversity of β-lactamases among *Enterobacteriaceae* in the nine U.S. census regions and ceftazidime-avibactam activity tested against isolates producing the most prevalent β-lactamase groups. Antimicrob Agents Chemother 2014;58:833–8.

28. Bowers JR, Kitchel B, Driebe EM, et al. Genomic analysis of the emergence and rapid global dissemination of the clonal group 258 *Klebsiella pneumoniae* pandemic. PLoS One 2015;10:e0133727.

29. Chen L, Mathema B, Chavda KD, et al. Carbapenemase-producing *Klebsiella pneumoniae*: molecular and genetic decoding. Trends Microbiol 2014;22: 686–96.

30. Dortet L, Poirel L, Nordmann P. Worldwide dissemination of the NDM-type carbapenemases in Gram-negative bacteria. Biomed Res Int 2014;2014:249856.

31. Qin S, Fu Y, Zhang Q, et al. High incidence and endemic spread of NDM-1-positive Enterobacteriaceae in Henan Province, China. Antimicrob Agents Chemother 2014;58:4275–82.

32. Rasheed JK, Kitchel B, Zhu W, et al. New Delhi metallo-β-lactamase-producing Enterobacteriaceae, United States. Emerg Infect Dis 2013;19:870–8.

33. Aitken SL, Tarrand JJ, Deshpande LM, et al. High rates of nonsusceptibility to ceftazidime-avibactam and identification of New Delhi metallo-β-lactamase production in Enterobacteriaceae bloodstream infections at a major cancer center. Clin Infect Dis 2016;63:954–8.

34. Pitout JD, Nordmann P, Poirel L. Carbapenemase-producing Klebsiella pneumoniae, a key pathogen set for global nosocomial dominance. Antimicrob Agents Chemother 2015;59:5873–84.

35. Anderson KF, Lonsway DR, Rasheed JK, et al. Evaluation of methods to identify the Klebsiella pneumoniae carbapenemase in Enterobacteriaceae. J Clin Microbiol 2007;45:2723–5.

36. Doyle D, Peirano G, Lascols C, et al. Laboratory detection of Enterobacteriaceae that produce carbapenemases. J Clin Microbiol 2012;50:3877–80.

37. van der Zwaluw K, de Haan A, Pluister GN, et al. The carbapenem inactivation method (CIM), a simple and low-cost alternative for the Carba NP test to assess phenotypic carbapenemase activity in gram-negative rods. PLoS One 2015;10: e0123690.

38. Tijet N, Patel SN, Melano RG. Detection of carbapenemase activity in Enterobacteriaceae: comparison of the carbapenem inactivation method versus the Carba NP test. J Antimicrob Chemother 2016;71:274–6.

39. Meini MR, Llarrull LI, Vila AJ. Overcoming differences: the catalytic mechanism of metallo-β-lactamases. FEBS Lett 2015;589:3419–32.

40. Franklin C, Liolios L, Peleg AY. Phenotypic detection of carbapenem-susceptible metallo-β-lactamase-producing gram-negative bacilli in the clinical laboratory. J Clin Microbiol 2006;44:3139–44.

41. Arakawa Y, Shibata N, Shibayama K, et al. Convenient test for screening metallo-β-lactamase-producing gram-negative bacteria by using thiol compounds. J Clin Microbiol 2000;38:40–3.

42. Beesley T, Gascoyne N, Knott-Hunziker V, et al. The inhibition of class C β-lactamases by boronic acids. Biochem J 1983;209:229–33.

43. Yagi T, Wachino J, Kurokawa H, et al. Practical methods using boronic acid compounds for identification of class C β-lactamase-producing Klebsiella pneumoniae and Escherichia coli. J Clin Microbiol 2005;43:2551–8.

44. Doi Y, Potoski BA, Adams-Haduch JM, et al. Simple disk-based method for detection of Klebsiella pneumoniae carbapenemase-type β-lactamase by use of a boronic acid compound. J Clin Microbiol 2008;46:4083–6.

45. Nordmann P, Poirel L, Dortet L. Rapid detection of carbapenemase-producing Enterobacteriaceae. Emerg Infect Dis 2012;18:1503–7.

46. Tijet N, Boyd D, Patel SN, et al. Evaluation of the Carba NP test for rapid detection of carbapenemase-producing Enterobacteriaceae and Pseudomonas aeruginosa. Antimicrob Agents Chemother 2013;57:4578–80.

47. Mirande C, Canard I, Buffet Croix Blanche S, et al. Rapid detection of carbapenemase activity: benefits and weaknesses of MALDI-TOF MS. Eur J Clin Microbiol Infect Dis 2015;34:2225–34.

48. Monteferrante CG, Sultan S, Ten Kate MT, et al. Evaluation of different pretreat-
    ment protocols to detect accurately clinical carbapenemase-producing Entero-
    bacteriaceae by MALDI-TOF. J Antimicrob Chemother 2016;71:2856–67.
49. Lasserre C, De Saint Martin L, Cuzon G, et al. Efficient detection of carbapenem-
    ase activity in *Enterobacteriaceae* by matrix-assisted laser desorption ionization-
    time of flight mass spectrometry in less than 30 minutes. J Clin Microbiol 2015;53:
    2163–71.
50. Oviano M, Sparbier K, Barba MJ, et al. Universal protocol for the rapid automated
    detection of carbapenem-resistant Gram-negative bacilli directly from blood cul-
    tures by matrix-assisted laser desorption/ionisation time-of-flight mass spectrom-
    etry (MALDI-TOF/MS). Int J Antimicrob Agents 2016;48(6):655–60.
51. Ledeboer NA, Lopansri BK, Dhiman N, et al. Identification of gram-negative bac-
    teria and genetic resistance determinants from positive blood culture broths by
    use of the Verigene Gram-negative blood culture multiplex microarray-based mo-
    lecular assay. J Clin Microbiol 2015;53:2460–72.
52. Hill JT, Tran KD, Barton KL, et al. Evaluation of the nanosphere Verigene BC-GN
    assay for direct identification of gram-negative bacilli and antibiotic resistance
    markers from positive blood cultures and potential impact for more-rapid anti-
    biotic interventions. J Clin Microbiol 2014;52:3805–7.
53. Salimnia H, Fairfax MR, Lephart PR, et al. Evaluation of the FilmArray blood cul-
    ture identification panel: results of a multicenter controlled trial. J Clin Microbiol
    2016;54:687–98.
54. Rand KH, Delano JP. Direct identification of bacteria in positive blood cultures:
    comparison of two rapid methods, FilmArray and mass spectrometry. Diagn Mi-
    crobiol Infect Dis 2014;79:293–7.
55. Tato M, Ruiz-Garbajosa P, Traczewski M, et al. Multisite evaluation of Cepheid
    Xpert Carba-R assay for detection of carbapenemase-producing organisms in
    rectal swabs. J Clin Microbiol 2016;54:1814–9.
56. Patel R. New developments in clinical bacteriology laboratories. Mayo Clin Proc
    2016;91:1448–59.
57. Doi Y, Paterson DL. Carbapenemase-producing Enterobacteriaceae. Semin Re-
    spir Crit Care Med 2015;36:74–84.
58. Tzouvelekis LS, Markogiannakis A, Piperaki E, et al. Treating infections caused by
    carbapenemase-producing Enterobacteriaceae. Clin Microbiol Infect 2014;20:
    862–72.
59. Gonzalez-Padilla M, Torre-Cisneros J, Rivera-Espinar F, et al. Gentamicin therapy
    for sepsis due to carbapenem-resistant and colistin-resistant *Klebsiella pneumo-
    niae*. J Antimicrob Chemother 2015;70:905–13.
60. Falcone M, Paterson D. Spotlight on ceftazidime/avibactam: a new option for
    MDR Gram-negative infections. J Antimicrob Chemother 2016;71:2713–22.
61. Shields RK, Potoski BA, Haidar G, et al. Clinical outcomes, drug toxicity and
    emergence of ceftazidime-avibactam resistance among patients treated for
    carbapenem-resistant *Enterobacteriaceae* infections. Clin Infect Dis 2016;
    63(12):1615–8.
62. Thaden JT, Pogue JM, Kaye KS. Role of newer and re-emerging older agents in
    the treatment of infections caused by carbapenem-resistant Enterobacteriaceae.
    Virulence 2016. [Epub ahead of print].
63. Kohira N, West J, Ito A, et al. *In vitro* antimicrobial activity of a siderophore ceph-
    alosporin, S-649266, against *Enterobacteriaceae* clinical isolates, including
    carbapenem-resistant strains. Antimicrob Agents Chemother 2016;60:729–34.

Tick-Borne Emerging Infections
Ehrlichiosis and Anaplasmosis

Nahed Ismail, MD, PhD, D(ABMM), D(ABMLI)[a],*, Jere W. McBride, PhD[b]

KEYWORDS

• Ehrlichiosis • Anaplasmosis • Pathogenesis • Immunity • Diagnosis

KEY POINTS

• Human ehrlichiosis and anaplasmosis are acute febrile tick-borne diseases caused by various members from the genera *Ehrlichia* and *Anaplasma*.

• Emerging infections with new *Ehrlichia* and *Anaplasma* species have become more frequently diagnosed as the cause of human infections, as animal reservoirs and tick vectors have increased in numbers and humans have inhabited areas where reservoir and tick populations are high.

• Human monocytotropic ehrlichiosis (HME) and human granulocytic anaplasmosis (HGA) have similar clinical presentations, including fever, headache, hematologic abnormalities (eg, leukopenia, and thrombocytopenia), and elevated liver enzymes.

• Neurologic manifestations are most frequently reported with HME.

OVERVIEW

Human ehrlichiosis and anaplasmosis are acute febrile tick-borne diseases caused by various members from the genera *Ehrlichia* and *Anaplasma*.[1–5] *Ehrlichia chaffeensis* is the major etiologic agent of human monocytotropic ehrlichiosis (HME), whereas *Anaplasma phagocytophilum* is the major cause of human granulocytic anaplasmosis (HGA). Emerging infections with new *Ehrlichia* and *Anaplasma* species have become more frequently diagnosed as the cause of human infections, as animal reservoirs and tick vectors have increased in numbers and humans have inhabited areas where reservoir and tick populations are high.

HME and HGA have similar clinical presentations, including fever, headache, hematologic abnormalities (eg, leukopenia and thrombocytopenia), and elevated liver

[a] Departments of Pathology and Immunology, School of Medicine, University of Pittsburgh, 3550 Terrace Street, Scaife Hall, Room 739, Pittsburgh, PA 15217, USA; [b] Department of Pathology, Center for Biodefense and Emerging Infectious Diseases, Sealy Center for Vaccine Development, University of Texas Medical Branch, 301 University Boulevard, Keiller 1.136, Galveston, TX 77555-0609, USA
* Corresponding author.
E-mail address: ismailn@upmc.edu

Clin Lab Med 37 (2017) 317–340
http://dx.doi.org/10.1016/j.cll.2017.01.006   labmed.theclinics.com
0272-2712/17/© 2017 Elsevier Inc. All rights reserved.

enzymes.[6–8] Symptoms typically begin a median of 9 days following a tick bite, with most patients seeking medical attention within the first 4 days of illness. Neurologic manifestations are most frequently reported with HME. This article reviews recent advances in the understanding of these rickettsial diseases as they relate to microbiology, epidemiology, diagnosis, pathogenesis, immunity, and treatment of the two prevalent tick-borne diseases found in the United States, HME and HGA.

MICROBIOLOGY

Ehrlichia and *Anaplasma* species are obligately intracellular alpha-proteobacteria that belong to the family Anaplasmataceae. The evolutionary relationships between these pathogens determined by the 16S ribosomal RNA gene (*rrs*) and GroEL comparisons indicate that *Ehrlichia* and *Anaplasma* spp share a common ancestor with other obligate intracellular pathogens, such as *Wolbachia*, *Neorickettsia*, *Orientia*, and *Rickettsia*.[9–12]

Ehrlichiosis

The *Ehrlichia* genus contains 7 named species: *E chaffeensis*, *E ewingii*, *E canis*, *E muris*, *E ruminantium*, *E ewingii*, and most recently *E mineirensis*, many of which are considered human zoonotic pathogens.[13–19] Human *E canis* infections in central and South America have been reported; however, it is primarily an important veterinary pathogen that naturally infects canids, causing canine monocytic ehrlichiosis and is transmitted by the brown dog tick, *Rhipicephalus sanguineus*.[20] Recently, an *E muris*–like agent (EMLA) has been identified as a new human pathogen in Minnesota and Wisconsin that is transmitted by *Ixodes scapularis*, contributing to geographically focused cases of EMLA HME in these northernmost states.[21–24]

Ehrlichia and *Anaplasma* species are small (approximately 0.4–1.5 μm) gram-negative bacteria that preferentially infect granulocytes *(A phagocytophilum* and *E ewingii)* or mononuclear phagocytes *(E chaffeensis*, *E canis*, and EMLA). They replicate within the host cytoplasmic vacuoles forming microcolonies called morulae, derived from the Latin word for mulberry. All *Ehrlichia* and *Anaplasma* species pathogenic for humans can be cultivated in cell culture except *E ewingii*.

Ehrlichia and *Anaplasma* species have the small genomes (0.8–1.5 Mb), which have been shaped by a reductive evolutionary processes that have resulted in dramatic gene loss and dependence on the host cell for survival.[19,25–28] *Ehrlichia* and *Anaplasma* exist intracellularly in 2 morphologically distinct ultrastructural forms: dense-cored cells (DCs) (0.4–0.6 μm) and reticulate cells (RCs) (0.4–0.6 μm by 0.7–1.9).[29–31] DCs are smaller and have an electron-dense chromatin, whereas the larger RCs have uniformly dispersed nucleoid filaments and ribosomes. *E chaffeensis* DCs and RCs can be distinguished by differentially expressed tandem repeat proteins (TRPs), TRP120 and TRP47.[32–35] DC forms are the infectious and trigger internalization into the host cell; within 24 hours after infection, DCs transform into RCs that begin dividing by binary fission. The full developmental cycle is complete by 72 hours, whereby RCs mature and become DCs and are released to infect other cells by undefined mechanisms.[29,36]

Ehrlichia and *Anaplasma* have the characteristic gram-negative cell wall structure but lack important cell membrane components, including lipopolysaccharide (LPS) and peptidoglycan.[37–39] LPS and peptidoglycan are 2 major pathogen-associated molecular patterns (PAMPS) that trigger innate responses during bacterial infection by binding to pattern recognition receptors (PRRs) of host cells.[40,41] Thus, the absence of these PAMPS seem to contribute to their evasion of innate host defense recognition. A recent study has demonstrated that *A phagocytophilum* exploits host cell cholesterol derived from the low-density lipoprotein receptor (LDLR)–mediated uptake pathway and LDLR regulatory system to accumulate cholesterol in their inclusions to facilitate replication.[42,43]

E chaffeensis, E ewingii, E canis, and *A phagocytophilum* have paralogous gene families that encode immunodominant outer membrane proteins (OMPs). These OMPs are members of Pfam PF01617 and constitute the OMP-1/MSP2/P44 family.[44–47] Evaluation of different *E chaffeensis* isolates revealed differential expression of OMP-1 members in infected macrophages and tick cell cultures.[48,49] In infected macrophages, the dominant *E chaffeensis* expressed OMPs are OMP-19 and OMP-20. In contract, OMP-14 is the only OMP expressed in cultured tick cells from the *E chaffeensis* tick vector (*Amblyomma americanum*) and EMLA and *A phagocytophilum* tick vector (*I scapularis*).[48–50] It is postulated that this differential expression of proteins within the OMP locus may be critical for adaptation of *Ehrlichia* species to their different hosts (mammals and ticks) possibly through their functional roles as porins.[44] Interestingly, vaccination with OMP-19 induced a strong humoral response and protected C57BL/6 mice from fatal *Ixodes ovatus* ehrlichia (IOE) infection, suggesting that expression of this protein in macrophages may contribute to induction of protective immunity against *Ehrlichia*.[47,51]

Ehrlichia have genes that encode type I and IV secretion systems, which are nanomachines that secrete effector proteins into the host cell.[3,52–54] Genes for the type IV secretion components are cotranscribed with genes for enzymes, such as superoxide dismutase, that catabolize reactive oxygen species. Several of the immunoreactive proteins of *E chaffeensis*, including ankyrin and TRPs, are type I secretion substrates.[34,54,55] TRPs are important effector proteins that interact with a diverse array of host proteins to modulate and activate host cell processes and are translocated to the host cell nucleus during infection.[33,34] All molecularly defined TRPs also contain major molecularly distinct linear B cell epitopes within the tandem repeat region that elicit strong species-specific antibody responses. Two TRPs (TRP120 and TRP47) are differentially expressed on DC ehrlichia, and both have been linked to the adhesion and internalization process via Wnt pathway activation.[56]

A phagocytophilum also has characterized effector proteins including AnkA and Ats-1 are both secreted by the type IV secretion system.[57–60] AnkA interacts with the host cell tyrosine kinase Abl and phosphotase SHP-1 in the cell cytoplasm and is also eventually transported into the host cell nucleus where it interacts with nuclear chromatin and seems to target gene regulatory regions.[28,35,55,61] Further comparison of ehrlichial genomes will provide insight and facilitate investigations of bacterial virulence factors, disease pathogenesis, and mechanisms of immune modulation and will provide targets for vaccines or new antimicrobial therapies.

EPIDEMIOLOGY
Human Monocytotropic Ehrlichiosis Epidemiology

The first case of HME was described in 1986, and HME became a reportable disease in 1994. The number of human ehrlichiosis cases reported to the Centers for Disease Control and Prevention (CDC) has steadily increased from less than 1 per million in 2000 to 3.4 per million in 2010.[7,62,63] However, this incidence is based on passive surveillance and likely is a significant underestimation of the actual disease incidence. Prospective studies in endemic areas have suggested rates of HME of 100 to 200 cases per million.[36,64] The true incidence of human infection with *E chaffeensis* is likely much higher because of underdiagnosis and underreporting. A seroprevalence study conducted among children residing in endemic areas found 20% had detectable antibody to E chaffeensis, without prior history of clinical disease.[65] However, because of cross-reactivity among Ehrlichia spp, it is impossible to conclude which of these patients were indeed infected with E chaffeensis.

Similar to other tick-borne diseases, the distribution of the arthropod vectors and vertebrate reservoirs correlates with the human disease incidence. States with the highest reported rates of HME include Missouri, Mississippi, Oklahoma, Tennessee, Arkansas, and Maryland. The dominant zoonotic cycle of E chaffeensis involves a reservoir of many persistently infected white-tailed deer (Odocoileus virginianus) and the tick vector, A americanum, prevalent throughout the Southeast and South Central United States. Other reservoirs, such as dogs and coyotes, and other tick vectors, including Ixodes pacificus, Ixodes ricinus, Amblyomma testudinarium, Amblyomma maculatum, and Dermacentor variabilis may also have a limited role in human transmission. Similar to other ticks, Amblyomma ticks have 3 feeding stages (larval, nymph, and adult). Each developmental stage feeds only once. Trans-stadial (ie, larva-nymph-adults) transmission of Ehrlichia occurs during nymph and adult feeding stages because larvae are uninfected. In contrast to Rickettsia spp, Ehrlichia are not maintained by transovarial transmission. The frequency of reported cases of HME is highest among males (incidence of 61%), people older than 50 years, and Caucasians. Although cases were reported year-round, the greatest number of cases occurred during the period of May through August, corresponding to periods of abundant tick populations and human outdoor recreation.

Epidemiology of Human Granulocytic Anaplasmosis

In the early 1990s, patients from Michigan and Wisconsin with a tick-bite history experiencing a febrile illness similar to HME were described.[66] These cases were distinguishable by the presence of inclusion bodies in granulocytes rather than monocytes, causing this syndrome initially to be referred to as human granulocytic ehrlichiosis.

The number of human anaplasmosis cases reported to the CDC has increased steadily since the disease became reportable, from 348 cases in 2000, to approximately 1800 cases in 2010. The incidence (the number of cases for every million persons) of anaplasmosis has also increased, from 1.4 cases per million persons in 2000 to 6.1 cases per million persons in 2010. However, the case fatality rate has remained low, at less than 1%.[62,67,68] The highest annual incidence rates of HGA in the United States have been reported in Connecticut (14–16 cases per 100,000), Wisconsin (24–58 cases per 100,000 population), and New York State (2.7 per 100,000).[62] Active surveillance in endemic areas has identified incidence rates of greater than 50 cases per 100,000 population.[69] As with E chaffeensis, sero-surveillance studies suggest that asymptomatic disease is common.[70] Demographic characteristics of patients with HGA are similar to patients with HME.

A phagocytophilum is transmitted by I scapularis in New England and North Central United States, I pacificus in the Western United States, I ricinus in Europe, and Ixodes persulcatus in Asia. Ixodes scapularis is also the tick vector for Borrelia burgdorferi, Babesia microti, and tick-borne encephalitis viruses; therefore, approximately 10% of patients with HGA have serologic evidence of coinfection with B burgdorferi or B microti.[71] The reservoir for A phagocytophilum is primarily small mammals, such as the white-footed mouse (Peromyscus leucopus), dusky-footed wood rats (Neotoma fuscipes), or others, such as Apodemus, Microtus, or Clethrionymus species, with humans serving as dead-end hosts.[72] Transmission of A phagocytophilum from a tick-mammalian reservoir and humans is similar to that of E chaffeensis. Cases occur year-round, with a peak incidence during June and July, perhaps reflecting the shorter arthropod season in these northern states or the relative importance of the nymphal stage of *Ixodes* ticks in disease transmission.

Epidemiology of Ehrlichiosis Ewingii

Ehrlichiosis ewingii was exclusively a canine pathogen, until a series of 4 human cases of *E ewingii* infection were described in 1999.[73] The epidemiology of HEE remains poorly defined because of the lack of a specific serologic assay for this organism and the absence of a dedicated reporting system for this infection. Most infections reported to date have occurred in patients with human immunodeficiency virus (HIV)[74] or who were immunosuppressed following organ transplantation.[75] *A americanum*, the primary vector for *E chaffeensis*, is also the primary vector for *E ewingii*. Most cases of HEE have been reported in Tennessee, Missouri, and Oklahoma. However, *E ewingii* infection in deer, dogs, and ticks has been described throughout the range of the lone star tick, suggesting that human infection with this pathogen might be more widespread than is currently documented.[72,76]

CLINICAL PRESENTATIONS
Human Monocytotropic Ehrlichiosis General Clinical Features

The clinical manifestations of HME and HGA are nonspecific and both are associated with similar flulike symptoms. Fever is an almost universal symptom (97%), followed by headaches (80%), myalgias (57%), and arthralgias (41%).[77] A skin eruption is relatively common among children with HME, occurring in 66% of pediatric cases compared with 21% of adults.[78,79] A rash is present in 10% of cases of HME and can be maculopapular, petechial, or characterized by diffuse erythroderma[80] but typically spares the face, palms, and soles. Nausea, vomiting, abdominal pain, and cough are variably present. Gastrointestinal symptoms, such as nausea, vomiting, diarrhea, anorexia, and abdominal pain, especially in children and pregnant women, are reported in patients with HME. Patients with HME can develop neurologic disorders, such as meningitis or meningoencephalitis. Central nervous system (CNS) involvement is identified in approximately 20% of patients with HME[81,82] and in some cases may be associated with seizures and coma.[74] Long-term neurologic sequelae in children are uncommon but include cognitive delays, fine motor impairment, and persistent foot drop.

HME is a more severe disease than HGA or HEE, with 62% of cases requiring hospitalization and a case-fatality rate of 3.7% as reported in 2003.[62] Up to 17% of patients develop life-threatening complications, although severe disease and death are more common in immunocompromised patients.[74] HME can be fatal in immunocompetent patients, whereby it presents as a multisystem disease resembling toxic or septic shock syndrome with multi-organ failure.[80,83] Other life-threatening manifestations include cardiovascular failure, aseptic meningitis, hemorrhages, hepatic insufficiency or failure, interstitial pneumonia, and adult respiratory distress syndrome.[5,36,84] The severity of the disease is greater in elderly and immunocompromised patients.

Although the clinical manifestations of *E chaffeensis* infection are nonspecific, laboratory abnormalities provide important diagnostic clues. A prospective cohort study of patients in an endemic area presenting with a febrile illness following a tick bite found a significantly lower white blood cell count (WBC) (mean 4.6×10^9 cells per liter) and neutrophil (mean 2.6×10^9 cells per liter) and platelet counts (mean 172×10^9 cells per liter) among patients with HME than noninfected patients,[78] and elevated transaminase levels were present in 83% of cases.[77] In pediatric patients, mild hyponatremia has been reported in 50% of the cases,[85] but this finding has been less frequently noted among infected adults. Among patients with HME with neurologic disorders, cerebrospinal fluid (CSF) pleocytosis is identified in approximately 60% of patients who undergo lumbar puncture whereby most samples have a lymphocytic predominance and a neutrophilic or mixed picture. The CSF WBC count is typically less than 100 cells per cubic millimeter, and protein may be mildly elevated. Morulae are rarely identified in CSF monocytes by Giemsa stain.[82,86] Radiographic imaging may be normal or may show leptomeningeal enhancement. Electroencephalogram may show nonspecific slowing.[82,87] Brain injury is limited, although atypical lymphoid infiltration of the leptomeninges and Virchow-Robin space with sparing of the brain parenchyma have been reported in one study.

Human Granulocytic Anaplasmosis General Clinical Features

HGA resembles HME with respect to the frequency of fever, headache, and myalgias; but rash is uncommon, noted in less than 10% of patients.[77] As with HME, leukopenia, thrombocytopenia, and elevations in transaminases are important clues to the diagnosis. HGA tends to be a less severe illness than HME, although life-threatening complications, including acute respiratory distress syndrome, acute renal failure, and hemodynamic collapse, have been reported.

Human Granulocytic Anaplasmosis Neurologic Features

CNS involvement is uncommon in HGA, with meningoencephalitis reported in only approximately 1% of cases.[77] In contrast, several different peripheral nervous system manifestations have been described, including brachial plexopathy, cranial nerve palsies, demyelinating polyneuropathy,[88] and bilateral facial nerve palsy. Recovery of neurologic function may be delayed over several months.[88] As the geographic distribution of *Borrelia burgdorferi* is similar to *Anaplasma phagocytophilum*, patients should be tested for coinfection because Lyme disease has similar neurologic manifestations. Although the cause of neurologic dysfunction in HGA is not yet known, it is thought to be due to complicating opportunistic infections or concomitant coinfection with *B burgdorferi*. Lumber puncture is performed less frequently for HGA than HME. Reported CSF abnormalities include lymphocytic pleocytosis and moderate elevation in protein.[89]

HEE General Clinical Features

Little is known of the clinical spectrum of HEE because of the paucity of reported cases. Symptoms seem to be similar to those described for HME and HGA. Despite the fact that most HEE infections have been in immunocompromised hosts, the clinical manifestations seem to be milder.[74,75] Findings of leukopenia, thrombocytopenia, and abnormal liver function tests are variably present.[73–75]

Headache is a frequent symptom in HEE and may be associated with meningitis, but the frequency of this finding and the spectrum of neurologic manifestations are unknown. One instance of neutrophilic pleocytosis in a patient with HEE has been reported.[73]

PATHOGENESIS AND IMMUNOPATHOLOGY
Human Monocytotropic Ehrlichiosis

Following a tick bite, *Ehrlichia chaffeensis* infects mononuclear phagocytes (monocytes/macrophages) and replicates by subverting host defense mechanisms. Recent studies have demonstrated that *E chaffeensis* exploits evolutionarily conserved host cell signaling pathways and host post-translational modification pathways to inhibit innate host defenses and interact with host cell target proteins in order to survive in the host cell.[37,90–93] Many molecular pathogen-host interactions have been defined that demonstrate the *E chaffeensis* effector interactions with a diverse array of host cell targets that control numerous host cell processes.[34,94,95] *E chaffeensis* enters the macrophages through receptor-mediated events that involve GPI-anchored surface receptors located within lipid rafts. Internalization via caveolae seems to be triggered by interactions of surface protein EtpE with the cell receptor deoxyribonuclease X as well as through interactions between TRPs and other surface receptors that likely include Wnt receptors.[56,96] Within the host cell, ehrlichia replicate in cytoplasmic vacuoles that resemble early endosomes that recruit a large array of host proteins.[33,34,97] *E chaffeensis* acquires nutrients by inducing autophagy activated by the type 4 effector, Etf-1.[98,99] Yet *E chaffeensis* also inhibits autophagolysosome generation by blocking lysosomal fusion through an unknown mechanism that seems to require effector proteins, whose expression is controlled by a 2-component regulatory system.[100,101]

Hijacking the host cell involves targeting of multiple cellular processes. It is now known that *E chaffeensis* has type 1 effectors (TRPs) that function in part as nucleomodulins, which bind host cell genes and reprogramming host cell gene expression (repression/activation) to favor survival. Globally, microarray analysis of THP-1 (human monocytic cell line) cells infected with *E chaffeensis* has revealed downregulation of T helper 1 (Th1) cytokines, such as interleukin (IL)-12 and IL-18, which are important inducers of adaptive Th1-mediated immune responses. *E chaffeensis* also downregulates genes, such as synaptosomal-associated protein, 23 kDa (SNAP 23), Rab5A (member of RAS oncogene family), and syntaxin 16 (STX16), which are involved in membrane trafficking, while upregulating apoptosis inhibitors and cell cyclins. *E chaffeensis* also circumvents host defenses by activating or inhibiting cell signaling pathways, including Wnt, Notch, and Jak/Stat (janus kinase/signal transducer and activator of transcription).[56,94,102,103] *E chaffeensis* also downregulates surface expression of toll-like receptors 2 and 4 and CD14 through TRP120 effector activation of the host cell Notch pathway (**Fig. 1**). The Notch pathway regulates PRR gene expression and inhibits activation of transcription factors that are involved in induction of proinflammatory innate immune responses.[94,104] Inhibition of Wnt, Notch, and PTM (post translational modification) pathways (SUMO [sumoylation]) results in ehrlichial destruction.[54,56,94] Studies using murine models of ehrlichiosis have demonstrated a pivotal role of TLR2 (toll like receptor-2) in induction of protective immune responses against ehrlichia and subsequent bacterial clearance.[105] In addition, ehrlichia lack LPS, which is the major ligand for TLR4. Thus, *Ehrlichia*-directed Notch activation resulting in downregulation of TLR2/4 and other Notch-regulated genes promotes survival of ehrlichia within the macrophage.[94]

Frequent pathologic findings of HME include granuloma formation, myeloid hyperplasia, and megakaryocytosis in the bone marrow.[106,107] Some patients develop erythrophagocytosis and plasmacytosis, suggesting a compensatory response.[108–110] Other pathologic findings in patients with severe HME include focal hepatocellular necrosis; hepatic granulomas; cholestasis; splenic and lymph node necrosis; diffuse mononuclear phagocyte hyperplasia of the spleen, liver, lymph node, and bone marrow; perivascular lymphohistiocytic infiltrates of various organs including kidney, heart, liver, meninges and brain; and interstitial mononuclear cell pneumonitis.[80,83,111] The severe pathology and multi-organ involvement in severe and fatal HME in immunocompetent patients is thought to be related to dysregulation of the host immune response that leads to tissue damage and eventually multisystem organ failure. This conclusion is based on the finding that in fatal disease in the form of toxic shock–like syndrome, uninfected hepatocytes undergo apoptosis without

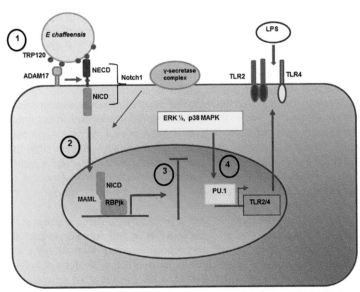

Fig. 1. Proposed model for *E chaffeensis* TRP120-mediated activation of canonical Notch signaling pathway and inhibition of TLR2/4 expression. (1) *E chaffeensis* TRP120 effector interaction with ADAM17 activates the metalloprotease resulting in cleavage of the substrate Notch1 and subsequent cleavage by γ-secretase causes (2) nuclear translocation of NICD (transcriptionally active intracellular domain), the transcriptionally active form that binds with RBPjκ and MAML proteins. (3) This triprotein complex activates transcription of Notch target genes, which causes inhibition of ERK1/2 and p38 MAPK pathway (4). The downstream transcription factor PU.1 expression is repressed, which causes further inhibition of monocyte TLR2/4 expression. Inhibition of TLR2/4 expression causes both inhibitions of *E chaffeensis* recognition and TLR-mediated proinflammatory cytokine production needed for the activation of monocytes and clearance of ehrlichia. ERK, extracellular signal-regulated kinases; MAML, mastermind-like protein 1; RBPJK, recombinant binding protein suppressor of hairless involved in NOTC signaling.

evidence of ehrlichial infection.[84,112,113] Similarly, analysis of hepatic tissues from autopsy cases in immunocompetent patients with HME showed that lymphohistiocytic foci, centrilobular and/or coagulation necrosis, Kupffer cell hyperplasia, and marked monocytic infiltration, *Ehrlichia*-infected cells are rarely identified.[113] In contrast, overwhelming ehrlichial burdens in the organs were observed in patients with HME who are immunocompromised because of other infections, such as HIV, or chemotherapy.[36,74] The hypothesis that severe and fatal *Ehrlichia*-induced toxic shock–like syndrome is due to an immunopathologic mechanism and is supported by studies in murine models of fatal ehrlichiosis whereby lethal ehrlichial infection with virulent *Ehrlichia* species named IOE results in a progressive, fatal ehrlichiosis that mimics toxic shock–like syndrome.[114–117] Characteristics of this syndrome/disease in these animals include liver injury and dysfunction marked by elevated liver enzymes (aspartate aminotransferase > alanine aminotransferase) and focal hepatic necrosis and apoptosis, significant leukopenia and lymphopenia mainly involving CD4+T lymphocytes and CD4+T cell apoptosis. Further analysis indicated that severe and fatal HME in animals is due to early overproduction of proinflammatory cytokines (eg, tumor necrosis factor [TNF]-α), and antiinflammatory IL-10 cytokines as well as chemokines, such as CCL2 (the chemokine [C-C motif] ligand 2). Interestingly, CD8+T cells seem to play a pathogenic role in HME whereby fatal disease is correlated with significant expansion of cytotoxic CD8+T cell producing TNF-α and interferon (IFN)-γ. Absence of CD8+T cells in animals infected with virulent *Ehrlichia* species protects against fatal disease, results in decreased tissue injury and normal CD4+T cell populations, and increases protective CD4+Th1 responses, suggesting that CD8+T-cell mediates lymphopenia and tissue damage in fatal HME in immunocompetent hosts. Consistent with the pathogenic role of CD8+T cells in fatal murine ehrlichiosis, Dierberg and Dumler[108] reported a significantly greater amount of hemophagocytosis (macrophage activation) and an increased number of CD8+ cells associated with low bacterial burden in the lymph nodes of patients who died of HME.[108,118]

Despite the extensive knowledge on adaptive immune responses against *Ehrlichia*, little is known about the innate immune signaling that lead to induction of host-pathogenic or protective immune responses. Recently, the authors have demonstrated that ehrlichia trigger activation of inflammasome,[105,119,120] a cytosolic multiprotein complexes that are triggered by PAMPs and damage-associated molecular patterns.[121,122] Activation of canonical inflammasome triggers cleavage of procaspase −1 into active caspase 1, which in turn induces the release of the cytokines IL-1β and IL-18 and inflammatory cell death known as pyroptosis.[123–125] Pyroptotic cell death is also mediated by active noncanonical caspase 11 in mice and caspase 4 in humans. The authors have recently showed that type I IFN receptor signaling is the master regulator of non–canonical inflammasome activation as it regulates caspase-11 activation and subsequent *Ehrlichia*-induced immunopathology in the liver.[105,119,120] These results were surprising as *Ehrlichia* lacks LPS, which is the prototypic cytosolic ligand that triggers activation of the non–canonical caspase-11 inflammasome during infection with gram-negative bacterial pathogens, such as *Salmonella*.

Studies with *E muris* have demonstrated that activation of innate lymphocytes, such as natural killer T cells (NKTs), occurs in a manner that is independent of TLRs but dependent on CD1d expression on antigen-presenting cells, such as dendritic cells.[126] Although NKT stimulation by *Ehrlichia* results in production of IFN-γ and elimination of intracellular ehrlichia, they also contribute to the development of *Ehrlichia*-induced toxic shock–like syndrome in murine models of fatal monocytic ehrlichiosis.[119,127–129]

Human Granulocytic Anaplasmosis

A phagocytophilum is observed predominantly in neutrophils in the peripheral blood and tissues from infected individuals. *A phagocytophilum* has the unique ability to selectively survive and multiply within cytoplasmic vacuoles of PMN (polymorphonuclear cells) cells by delaying their apoptosis through upregulation of antiapoptotic bcl-2 (B-cell lymphoma 2) family member bfl-1 and blocking FAS (CD95)–induced programmed cell death of human neutrophils.[130–132] *A phagocytophilum* uses multiple evasion strategies to inhibit neutrophil antimicrobial functions. Some studies have suggested that one of the mechanisms by which *A phagocytophilum* avoids the toxic effects of neutrophils is its ability to inhibit the fusion of the lysosomes with the cytoplasmic vacuoles and by arresting or inhibiting other signaling pathways related to respiratory burst.[61,133,134] *A phagocytophilum* seems to modulate host cell gene transcription through AnkA, a secreted type IV effector protein that is transported to the infected host cell nucleus through binding to host target genes, such as *cybb*.[55,58,59] Further studies are required to establish the effects of AnkA binding on neutrophil functions. The molecular basis by which *A phagocytophilum* affects respiratory burst of granulocytes shown to be due to the downregulation of gp91[phox] and rac2, 2 important components of nicotinamide adenine dinucleotide phosphate oxidase.[135] Paradoxically, another study showed that infection with *A phagocytophilum* induced protracted degranulation in human neutrophils, which was attributed to inflammatory tissue injury. In addition, *A phagocytophilum* upregulates the production of the chemokine IL-8 as well as proinflammatory cytokines, which may account for enhanced recruitment of neutrophils and tissue injury. Recently, a novel inflammasome complex (NLRC4 [nod-like receptor family-card domain -containing protein 4]) pathway was described that depends on the prostaglandin E2 (PGF2) and the EP3 receptor.[136] These results are surprising, as *Anaplasma* does not express flagellin, which is the typical PAMP for NLRC4.[137,138]

Pathologic findings in patients with HGA and animal models include normocellular or hypercellular bone marrow, erythrophagocytosis, hepatic apoptosis and periportal lymphohistiocytic infiltrates focal splenic necrosis, and mild interstitial pneumonitis and pulmonary hemorrhage.[55,139–142] Similar to HME, HGA hematologic abnormalities include marked leukopenia and thrombocytopenia. Although the immune mechanisms that account for severe and fatal HGA are not completely understood, there is some evidence of immunosuppression in patients with HGA.[143] This conclusion is supported by the high number of fatal cases due to secondary opportunistic infections and organ failures. The mechanism by which this immune suppression occurs in HGA is not yet defined.

REINFECTION AND IMMUNITY
Human Monocytotropic Ehrlichiosis

Immunity to primary *E chaffeensis* infection in humans has not been investigated, but comparative murine models have provided some insight. A role for cell-mediated immunity has been suggested based on the severity of *E chaffeensis* infection in HIV-infected patients and the lymphoproliferative responses observed in patients following recovery from HME.[36] However, the relative importance of cell-mediated and humoral immunity has not been firmly established. Studies using murine models have suggested that protective immunity during primary and secondary ehrlichial infection is mediated by cellular immunity, mainly CD4$^+$ T cells producing IFN-γ (ie, Th1 cells).[47,51,116,144,145] IFN-γ production by CD4+Th1 cells likely leads to macrophage activation and induction of bactericidal mechanisms, such as production of reactive oxygen species, which in turn leads to bacterial elimination. In addition to IFN-γ, murine studies have shown that proinflammatory cytokines, such as IL-12p40 and TNF-γ, are also important factors in clearance of *Ehrlichia* and protection.[114,115,146,147] Humoral immunity seems to also play a role in protection against *Ehrlichia* infection as evidenced by significant seroconversion in patients who recover from disease.[148,149] In murine studies, *Ehrlichia*-specific antibodies, mainly immunoglobulin G2a (IgG2a) (Th1-dependent Ig subclass), protect severe combined immunodeficiency mice from severe *Ehrlichia chaffeensis* infection.[147,150–153]

It is unknown whether patients who recovered from HME are immune or susceptible to reinfection. Such evidence is limited to a single report of reinfection with a genetically distinct *E chaffeensis* strain in a liver transplant recipient receiving immunosuppressive therapy.[154] In murine studies, the development of heterologous protection model of ehrlichiosis has provided a mechanism to investigate immunity, including memory immune responses.[114,116] These studies indicate that prior infection of immunocompetent mice with *E muris* that cause persistent asymptomatic infection in mice and strong cell-mediated immune responses protect against secondary infection with highly virulent *Ehrlichia* species (IOE) that cause fatal disease in uninfected hosts. Heterologous protection against *Ehrlichia* is associated with minimal tissue injury, development of well-defined granulomas, expansion of IFN-g producing effector memory

CD4+ and CD8+type-1 cells, and substantial production of *Ehrlichia*-specific IgG2a antibodies. Vaccines are currently unavailable for HME.

Human Granulocytic Anaplasmosis

Currently, little is known about immunity following an *A phagocytophilum* infection. Although infection may result in long-term immunity, there have been rare reports of laboratory-confirmed reinjection. Thus, individuals who live in endemic areas and are at risk of exposure to infected ticks should be vigilant about avoiding tick bites and other tick-borne pathogens. Similar to immunity against *E chaffeensis*, protective immunity against *A phagocytophilum* is mediated by cellular and humoral immune mechanisms. It is generally thought that individuals who develop high titer antibodies are protected against reinfection; patients previously infected with *A phagocytophilum* develop high titer antibodies that may last for as long as 3 years. Whether this persistence of antibodies is due to persistent infection or reinfection is not clearly determined. Similarly, it is not known if previous infection of humans leads to antigen-specific memory T- and B-cell responses that protect individuals against reinfection. Vaccines are currently unavailable for HGA.

DIAGNOSIS OF HUMAN MONOCYTOTROPIC EHRLICHIOSIS AND HUMAN GRANULOCYTIC ANAPLASMOSIS

Diagnosis of HME and HGA rests primarily on clinical suspicion because of the limited availability of rapid diagnostic tests, such as polymerase chain reaction (PCR), and the absence of detectable serum antibodies at the time of clinical presentation (4 days after the onset of clinical illness).[155–158] The prognosis worsens if treatment is not administered or delayed[109]; therefore, it is important that empirical therapy with doxycycline be started for any patient with compatible clinical and laboratory findings. Initial diagnosis of ehrlichiosis can be based on nonspecific biochemical and hematologic findings. However, confirmatory tests should be performed at different intervals after the onset of illness.

HEMATOLOGIC AND BIOCHEMICAL ABNORMALITIES

Presumptive diagnosis of HME and HGA is based on clinical manifestation; clues from medical history, such as history of tick bite and outdoor activities; as well as specific laboratory abnormalities. Pancytopenia is a hallmark laboratory feature of HME early in the course of the illness. Anemia occurs within 2 weeks of illness and influences 50% of patients.[159,160] Mild to moderate leukopenia with largest decline in lymphocyte population is observed in approximately 60% to 70% of patients during the first week of illness.[4,112] Interestingly, during convalescence, a significant increase in lymphocyte count, that is, relative and absolute lymphocytosis, is seen in most patients and is characterized predominantly by the expansion of activated $\gamma\delta$ T cells.[161,162] Marked thrombocytopenia is one of pathognomonic findings in HME, which is usually detected in 70% to 90% of patients during their illness. Mildly or moderately elevated hepatic transaminase levels are detected in approximately 90% of patients associated with increased levels of alkaline phosphatase and bilirubin in some patients. Mild to moderate hyponatremia has been reported in as many as 50% of adult patients and 70% of pediatric patients.

Other laboratory abnormalities that occur in severe disease are specific to the organ involved. Examples are increased serum creatinine, lactate dehydrogenase, creatine phosphokinase, amylase, and electrolyte abnormalities, including hypocalcemia, hypomagnesemia, hypophosphatemia, prolonged prothrombin times, increased levels of fibrin degradation products, metabolic acidosis, profound hypotension, disseminated intravascular coagulopathy, hepatic and renal failure, adrenal insufficiency, and myocardial dysfunction.[1,163]

SPECIFIC LABORATORY DIAGNOSTIC TESTS

A diagnosis of HME and HGA can be confirmed by several laboratory methods.[164,165] These tests include serologic detection of specific antibodies, detection of morulae in peripheral blood or in CSF leukocytes, detection of ehrlichial DNA by PCR of blood or CSF, direct detection of ehrlichia in tissue samples by immunohistochemistry, and isolation of bacteria.

SEROLOGIC TESTING

Serologic testing of IgM and IgG antibodies specific to *E chaffeensis* or *A phagocytophilum* using indirect immunofluorescence assay (IFA) is the gold standard and is the most frequently used confirmatory test for HME. Paired sera collected during a 3- to 6-week interval represent the preferred specimens for serologic evaluation of HME. Diagnosis of HME will be made when any of the following serology results are obtained: a) a single IgG antibody titer of at least 256; b) seroconversion from negative to positive antibody status with a minimum titer of 64; c) a four-fold increase in titer during convalescence. Although serology is one of major diagnostic criterion for ehrlichiosis, it has several limitations that should be considered: (1) The IgG IFA test is negative in as many as 80% of patients during the first week of illness, and the IgM titers may also be uninformative at this time; thus, a negative serologic results for the acute-phase sample does not exclude the diagnosis. (2) A high rate of false-positive serology usually occurs because of cross-reactive antigens shared by *Ehrlichia* and *Anaplasma* that induce cross-reactive antibodies. Because of this cross-reactivity among ehrlichial species, sera should be tested against both *E chaffeensis* and *A phagocytophilum* antigens when ascribing a specific cause. (3) Failure to seroconvert, in some cases, can be attributed to immune impairment. (4) Early treatment with a tetracycline-class antibiotics occasionally reduces or abrogates the antibody response to *E chaffeensis*.

BLOOD SMEAR STAINING

Diagnosis of HME and HGA can be accomplished by staining of blood smears from peripheral blood, bone marrow, or CSF to detect morulae. Smears can be stained with Wright, Diff-Quik, or Giemsa stains. Although this method is rapid, it is relatively insensitive compared with other confirmatory tests, especially in immunocompetent patients whereby severe disease is usually associated with very low bacterial burden in blood and peripheral organs. Morulae are detected within monocytes in only about 3% of patients with HME. In contrast, blood smear is more useful for HGA diagnosis, as 25% to 75% of patients have morulae in peripheral blood examinations and sensitivity is highest during the first week of infection.

POLYMERASE CHAIN REACTION AMPLIFICATION

Because of its high specificity (60%–85%) and sensitivity (60%–85% for *E chaffeensis* and 67%–90% for *A phagocytophilum*) as well as rapid turnaround time, diagnosis of ehrlichial infection by PCR has become the test of choice for confirming serology indicating HME and HGA. PCR is the only definitive diagnostic test for *E ewingii* infection because the bacteria is uncultivable, although the sensitivity and specificity of this approach is unknown. Multiplex or multicolor testing capable of detecting several related etiologic agents has been described.[157] PCR of whole blood is commercially available and allows rapid diagnosis of infection in up to 85% of cases.[166] Blood samples should be collected in ethylenediaminetetraacetic acid or sodium citrate anticoagulants and obtained before or at the initiation of therapy to increase sensitivity. However, because doxycycline treatment is effective only at early stages of infection, treatment should start as soon as possible while waiting for laboratory results. PCR detection is particularly important for detection of ehrlichial infection at early stages when antibody levels are very low or undetectable. Although PCR of CSF may be positive, the sensitivity is lower than for whole blood, likely because of the significantly lower volume of infected cells.[167] Several PCR targets have been used among different *Ehrlichia* isolates including the *rrs* (16S rRNA) and *groESL* heat shock operon. Other genes have been used, such as the genus-specific disulfide bond formation protein gene, the *E chaffeensis*-specific 120-kDa and TRP32 protein (VLPT [variable-length PCR target]) genes, and the 28-kDa OMP-p28.

ISOLATION

Similar to other infectious diseases, cultivation of *Ehrlichia* and *Anaplasma* is the gold standard in diagnosis of HME and HGA. However, primary isolation may take up to several weeks. The sensitivity of *E chaffeensis* isolation compared with PCR amplification is very low. In contrast, the sensitivity of culture for detection of *A phagocytophilum* can be equivalent to that of PCR and blood smear examination. Similar to PCR amplification and blood smear examination, prior doxycycline treatment diminishes the sensitivity of culture to a greater degree. Because of the lower sensitivity of this method, therapeutic decisions must often be based on a high index of clinical suspicion and laboratory evidence of the infection, such as PCR assays and peripheral blood smears.

IMMUNOHISTOCHEMISTRY

Immunohistochemical staining of the formalin fixed biopsy or autopsy tissues is another confirmatory method for diagnosis of *Ehrlichia* and *Anaplasma* infection. The immunohistochemistry method is most useful in documenting the presence of organisms in patients before initiation of antibiotic therapy or within the first 48 hours after antibiotic therapy has been initiated. IHC techniques are also available for diagnosing cases of ehrlichiosis and anaplasmosis from bone marrow biopsies and tissue obtained at autopsy of fatal cases, including the spleen, lymph nodes, liver, and lung.

HEE DIAGNOSIS

A diagnosis of HEE is suggested by visualization of intracytoplasmic morulae in neutrophils in patients with residence or travel to an area of HME (rather than HGA) endemicity. Morulae may be visualized in both blood and, rarely, CSF.[73] Although there is no specific serologic assay for *E ewingii*, there is significant serologic cross-reactivity to *E chaffeenesis*.[73] It is conceivable that in the absence of visualization of morulae in granulocytes or confirmatory PCR for *E ewingii*, a proportion of cases meeting serologic criteria for HME actually represent HEE infection. A specific PCR for *E ewingii* exists but is limited to research laboratories. Similar to the PCR for *E chaffeensis* and *A phagocytophilum*, sensitivity is maximal early in the course of the illness, before antibiotic therapy.

DIFFERENTIAL DIAGNOSIS

The differential diagnosis of HME, HGA, and HEE at early stages of the disease whereby the symptoms and signs of disease are nonspecific and patients present with fever, headache, myalgia, and malaise may include various viral syndromes, Rocky Mountain spotted fever, upper respiratory illness, urinary tract infection, and sepsis. If history of a tick bite and outdoor activities exist with these symptoms, the physician should consider other tick-borne febrile illnesses, such as Rocky Mountain spotted fever, relapsing fever, tularemia, Lyme borreliosis, Colorado tick fever, and babesiosis. CNS signs and symptoms with CSF pleocytosis suggest viral or bacterial meningoencephalitis.[81,82,159] Other diseases that share clinical and laboratory findings of ehrlichial disease, particularly if patients presented with rash, are meningococcemia, toxic shock syndrome, murine typhus, Q fever, typhoid fever, leptospirosis, hepatitis, enteroviral infection, influenza, bacterial sepsis, endocarditis, Kawasaki disease, collagen-vascular diseases, and immune thrombocytopenic purpura.

TREATMENT

In vitro susceptibility testing has shown that E chaffeensis is resistant to representatives of most classes of antibiotics, including aminoglycosides (gentamicin), fluoroquinolones (ciprofloxacin), penicillins (penicillin), macrolides and ketolides (erythromycin and telithromycin), and sulfa-containing drugs (cotrimoxazole).[155,164,168,169] Chloramphenicol is an alternative drug that has been considered for treatment of HGA or HME. However, this drug is associated with various side effects and might require monitoring of blood indices; therefore, it is no longer available in the oral form in the United States.

Doxycycline is the recommended treatment of HME; the adult dosage is 100 mg orally twice daily, and the pediatric dosage for children less than 100 lb (45.4 kg) is 2.2 mg/kg twice daily. Response to treatment is typically rapid, and fever persisting greater than 72 hours after initiation of treatment strongly suggests an alternative diagnosis. The recommended dosage is 100 mg per dose administered twice daily (orally or intravenously) for adults or 2.2 mg/kg body weight per dose administered twice daily (orally or intravenously) for children weighing less than 100 lb (45.4 kg). Although no studies have specifically addressed the duration of treatment, most authorities advocate continuing antibiotics for 3 to 5 days after defervescence[72] and perhaps longer (eg, total of 10–14 days) if there is CNS involvement.[81] During pregnancy, doxycycline is contraindicated; successful treatment with rifampin has been reported and can be an effective alternative.[2]

HUMAN GRANULOCYTIC ANAPLASMOSIS TREATMENT

Therapeutic considerations for HGA are similar to HME, with doxycycline remaining the drug of choice for both pediatric and adult cases. If coinfection with Borrelia burgdorferi is suspected based on characteristic skin findings or elevated antibodies, doxycycline should be continued for at least 10 days for adults.[169] In B burgdorferi coinfected children less than 8 years of age, doxycycline should be continued until patients are afebrile for 3 days, with the remainder of the 14-day course completed with an alternative agent active against B burgdorferi (eg, amoxicillin or cefuroxime axetil) to minimize the risk of dental discoloration.[77] Patients who fail to respond clinically to doxycycline monotherapy after 72 hours should be evaluated for an alternative diagnosis or the possibility of Babesia coinfection.

PREVENTION

Preventive antibiotic therapy for ehrlichial infection is not indicated for patients who have had recent tick bites and are not ill. Avoidance of tick bites and immediate removal of ticks remains the ultimate prevention approach. Individuals who live in endemic areas should wear light-colored clothes during outdoor activities, which allows individuals to see crawling ticks. Adults who are at high risk of getting bitten by ticks should apply chemoprophylactic repellents, such as n, n-diethyl-m-toluamide to exposed skin that prevents tick attachment as they repel the ticks. Individuals should carefully inspect their bodies, hair, and clothes on return from potentially tick-infested areas for ticks and should immediately remove any attached tick. Studies have shown that a period of 4 to 24 hours of attachment of infected ticks to the host may be required before effective transmission of *Ehrlichia* and *Anaplasma* to occur. Therefore, immediate and complete removal of attached ticks is critical for prevention of transmission and infection.

REFERENCES

1. Bakken JS, Krueth J, Wilson-Nordskog C, et al. Clinical and laboratory characteristics of human granulocytic ehrlichiosis. JAMA 1996;275:199–205.

2. Cheng Z, Kumagai Y, Lin M, et al. Intra-leukocyte expression of two-component systems in Ehrlichia chaffeensis and Anaplasma phagocytophilum and effects of the histidine kinase inhibitor closantel. Cell Microbiol 2006;8:1241–52.

3. Rikihisa Y. Molecular events involved in cellular invasion by Ehrlichia chaffeensis and Anaplasma phagocytophilum. Vet Parasitol 2010;167:155–66.

4. Olano JP, Hogrefe W, Seaton B, et al. Clinical manifestations, epidemiology, and laboratory diagnosis of human monocytotropic ehrlichiosis in a commercial laboratory setting. Clin Diagn Lab Immunol 2003;10:891–6.

5. Alcantara VE, Gallardo EG, Hong C, et al. Typhus group Rickettsiae antibodies in rural Mexico. Emerg Infect Dis 2004;10:549–51.

6. Rikihisa Y. Clinical and biological aspects of infection caused by Ehrlichia chaffeensis. Microbes Infect 1999;1:367–76.

7. Dumler JS, Madigan JE, Pusterla N, et al. Ehrlichioses in humans: epidemiology, clinical presentation, diagnosis, and treatment. Clin Infect Dis 2007;45(Suppl 1): S45–51.

8. Ismail N, Walker DH. Balancing protective immunity and immunopathology: a unifying model of monocytotropic ehrlichiosis. Ann N Y Acad Sci 2005;1063: 383–94.

9. Dumler JS, Barbet AF, Bekker CP, et al. Reorganization of genera in the families Rickettsiaceae and Anaplasmataceae in the order Rickettsiales: unification of some species of Ehrlichia with Anaplasma, Cowdria with Ehrlichia and Ehrlichia with Neorickettsia, descriptions of six new species combinations and designation of Ehrlichia equi and 'HGE agent' as subjective synonyms of Ehrlichia phagocytophila. Int J Syst Evol Microbiol 2001;51:2145–65.

10. Ohashi N, Unver A, Zhi N, et al. Cloning and characterization of multigenes encoding the immunodominant 30-kilodalton major outer membrane proteins of Ehrlichia canis and application of the recombinant protein for serodiagnosis. J Clin Microbiol 1998;36:2671–80.

11. Zhang Y, Ohashi N, Lee EH, et al. Ehrlichia sennetsu groE operon and antigenic properties of the GroEL homolog. FEMS Immunol Med Microbiol 1997;18:39–46.

12. Kumagai Y, Cheng Z, Lin M, et al. Biochemical activities of three pairs of Ehrlichia chaffeensis two-component regulatory system proteins involved in inhibition of lysosomal fusion. Infect Immun 2006;74:5014–22.

13. Aguiar DM, Ziliani TF, Zhang X, et al. A novel Ehrlichia genotype strain distinguished by the TRP36 gene naturally infects cattle in Brazil and causes clinical manifestations associated with ehrlichiosis. Ticks Tick Borne Dis 2014;5:537–44.

14. Cabezas-Cruz A, Zweygarth E, Vancova M, et al. Ehrlichia minasensis sp. nov., a new species within the genus Ehrlichia isolated from the tick Rhipicephalus microplus. Int J Syst Evol Microbiol 2016. [Epub ahead of print].

15. Jahfari S, Hofhuis A, Fonville M, et al. Molecular detection of tick-borne pathogens in humans with tick bites and erythema migrans, in The Netherlands. PLoS Negl Trop Dis 2016;10:e0005042.

16. Allen MB, Pritt BS, Sloan LM, et al. First reported case of Ehrlichia ewingii involving human bone marrow. J Clin Microbiol 2014;52:4102–4.

17. Liebenberg J, Pretorius A, Faber FE, et al. Identification of Ehrlichia ruminantium proteins that activate cellular immune responses using a reverse vaccinology strategy. Vet Immunol Immunopathol 2012;145:340–9.

18. Felek S, Greene R, Rikihisa Y. Transcriptional analysis of p30 major outer membrane protein genes of Ehrlichia canis in naturally infected ticks and sequence analysis of p30-10 of E canis from diverse geographic regions. J Clin Microbiol 2003;41:886–8.

19. Thirumalapura NR, Qin X, Kuriakose JA, et al. Complete genome sequence of ehrlichia muris strain AS145T, a model monocytotropic ehrlichia strain. Genome Announc 2014;2(1):e01234–13.

20. Unvera A, Rikihisa Y, Karaman M, et al. An acute severe ehrlichiosis in a dog experimentally infected with a new virulent strain of Ehrlichia canis. Clin Microbiol Infect 2009;15(Suppl 2):59–61.

21. Saito TB, Thirumalapura NR, Shelite TR, et al. An animal model of a newly emerging human ehrlichiosis. J Infect Dis 2015;211:452–61.

22. Saito TB, Walker DH. A tick vector transmission model of monocytotropic ehrlichiosis. J Infect Dis 2015;212(6):968–77.

23. Pritt BS, Sloan LM, Johnson DK, et al. Emergence of a new pathogenic Ehrlichia species, Wisconsin and Minnesota, 2009. N Engl J Med 2011;365:422–9.

24. Castillo CG, Eremeeva ME, Paskewitz SM, et al. Detection of human pathogenic Ehrlichia muris-like agent in Peromyscus leucopus. Ticks Tick Borne Dis 2015;6: 155–7.

25. Cheng C, Nair AD, Indukuri VV, et al. Targeted and random mutagenesis of Ehrlichia chaffeensis for the identification of genes required for in vivo infection. PLoS Pathog 2013;9:e1003171.

26. Dunning Hotopp JC, Lin M, Madupu R, et al. Comparative genomics of emerging human ehrlichiosis agents. PLoS Genet 2006;2:e21.

27. Brayton KA, Palmer GH, Brown WC. Genomic and proteomic approaches to vaccine candidate identification for Anaplasma marginale. Expert Rev Vaccines 2006;5:95–101.

28. Felek S, Huang H, Rikihisa Y. Sequence and expression analysis of virB9 of the type IV secretion system of Ehrlichia canis strains in ticks, dogs, and cultured cells. Infect Immun 2003;71:6063–7.

29. Zhang JZ, Popov VL, Gao S, et al. The developmental cycle of Ehrlichia chaffeensis in vertebrate cells. Cell Microbiol 2007;9:610–8.

30. Popov VL, Korenberg EI, Nefedova VV, et al. Ultrastructural evidence of the ehrlichial developmental cycle in naturally infected Ixodes persulcatus ticks in the

course of coinfection with Rickettsia, Borrelia, and a flavivirus. Vector Borne Zoonotic Dis 2007;7:699–716.

31. Luo T, Zhang X, Wakeel A, et al. A variable-length PCR target protein of Ehrlichia chaffeensis contains major species-specific antibody epitopes in acidic serine-rich tandem repeats. Infect Immun 2008;76:1572–80.

32. Kuriakose JA, Zhang X, Luo T, et al. Molecular basis of antibody mediated immunity against Ehrlichia chaffeensis involves species-specific linear epitopes in tandem repeat proteins. Microbes Infect 2012;14:1054–63.

33. Luo T, Kuriakose JA, Zhu B, et al. Ehrlichia chaffeensis TRP120 interacts with a diverse array of eukaryotic proteins involved in transcription, signaling, and cytoskeleton organization. Infect Immun 2011;79:4382–91.

34. Luo T, McBride JW. Ehrlichia chaffeensis TRP32 interacts with host cell targets that influence intracellular survival. Infect Immun 2012;80:2297–306.

35. Luo T, Zhang X, Nicholson WL, et al. Molecular characterization of antibody epitopes of Ehrlichia chaffeensis ankyrin protein 200 and tandem repeat protein 47 and evaluation of synthetic immunodeterminants for serodiagnosis of human monocytotropic ehrlichiosis. Clin Vaccine Immunol 2010;17:87–97.

36. Walker DH. Ehrlichia under our noses and no one notices. Arch Virol Suppl 2005;19:147–56.

37. Rikihisa Y. Anaplasma phagocytophilum and Ehrlichia chaffeensis: subversive manipulators of host cells. Nat Rev Microbiol 2010;8:328–39.

38. Huang H, Lin M, Wang X, et al. Proteomic analysis of and immune responses to Ehrlichia chaffeensis lipoproteins. Infect Immun 2008;76:3405–14.

39. Lin M, Rikihisa Y. Ehrlichia chaffeensis and Anaplasma phagocytophilum lack genes for lipid A biosynthesis and incorporate cholesterol for their survival. Infect Immun 2003;71:5324–31.

40. Lupfer C, Kanneganti TD. The expanding role of NLRs in antiviral immunity. Immunol Rev 2013;255:13–24.

41. Broz P, Monack DM. Molecular mechanisms of inflammasome activation during microbial infections. Immunol Rev 2011;243:174–90.

42. Klionsky DJ, Abdalla FC, Abeliovich H, et al. Guidelines for the use and interpretation of assays for monitoring autophagy. Autophagy 2012;8:445–544.

43. Xiong Q, Lin M, Rikihisa Y. Cholesterol-dependent anaplasma phagocytophilum exploits the low-density lipoprotein uptake pathway. PLoS Pathog 2009;5:e1000329.

44. Kumagai Y, Huang H, Rikihisa Y. Expression and porin activity of P28 and OMP-1F during intracellular Ehrlichia chaffeensis development. J Bacteriol 2008;190:3597–605.

45. Lin M, Kikuchi T, Brewer HM, et al. Global proteomic analysis of two tick-borne emerging zoonotic agents: Anaplasma phagocytophilum and ehrlichia chaffeensis. Front Microbiol 2011;2:24.

46. Lin Q, Rikihisa Y, Felek S, et al. Anaplasma phagocytophilum has a functional msp2 gene that is distinct from p44. Infect Immun 2004;72:3883–9.

47. Crocquet-Valdes PA, Thirumalapura NR, Ismail N, et al. Immunization with Ehrlichia P28 outer membrane proteins confers protection in a mouse model of ehrlichiosis. Clin Vaccine Immunol 2011;18:2018–25.

48. Peddireddi L, Cheng C, Ganta RR. Promoter analysis of macrophage- and tick cell-specific differentially expressed Ehrlichia chaffeensis p28-Omp genes. BMC Microbiol 2009;9:99.

49. Singu V, Peddireddi L, Sirigireddy KR, et al. Unique macrophage and tick cell-specific protein expression from the p28/p30-outer membrane protein multigene

locus in Ehrlichia chaffeensis and Ehrlichia canis. Cell Microbiol 2006;8: 1475–87.

50. Ganta RR, Cheng C, Miller EC, et al. Differential clearance and immune responses to tick cell-derived versus macrophage culture-derived Ehrlichia chaffeensis in mice. Infect Immun 2007;75:135–45.

51. Nandi B, Hogle K, Vitko N, et al. CD4 T-cell epitopes associated with protective immunity induced following vaccination of mice with an ehrlichial variable outer membrane protein. Infect Immun 2007;75:5453–9.

52. Liu H, Bao W, Lin M, et al. Ehrlichia type IV secretion effector ECH0825 is translocated to mitochondria and curbs ROS and apoptosis by upregulating host MnSOD. Cell Microbiol 2012;14:1037–50.

53. Bao W, Kumagai Y, Niu H, et al. Four VirB6 paralogs and VirB9 are expressed and interact in Ehrlichia chaffeensis-containing vacuoles. J Bacteriol 2009; 191:278–86.

54. Dunphy PS, Luo T, McBride JW. Ehrlichia chaffeensis exploits host SUMOylation pathways to mediate effector-host interactions and promote intracellular survival. Infect Immun 2014;82:4154–68.

55. Centers for Disease Control and Prevention (CDC). Anaplasma phagocytophilum transmitted through blood transfusion–Minnesota, 2007. MMWR Morb Mortal Wkly Rep 2008;57:1145–8.

56. Luo T, Dunphy PS, Lina TT, et al. Ehrlichia chaffeensis exploits canonical and noncanonical host Wnt signaling pathways to stimulate phagocytosis and promote intracellular survival. Infect Immun 2015;84:686–700.

57. Lin M, den Dulk-Ras A, Hooykaas PJ, et al. Anaplasma phagocytophilum AnkA secreted by type IV secretion system is tyrosine phosphorylated by Abl-1 to facilitate infection. Cell Microbiol 2007;9:2644–57.

58. Lockwood S, Voth DE, Brayton KA, et al. Identification of Anaplasma marginale type IV secretion system effector proteins. PLoS One 2011;6:e27724.

59. Park J, Kim KJ, Choi KS, et al. Anaplasma phagocytophilum AnkA binds to granulocyte DNA and nuclear proteins. Cell Microbiol 2004;6:743–51.

60. Scharf W, Schauer S, Freyburger F, et al. Distinct host species correlate with Anaplasma phagocytophilum ankA gene clusters. J Clin Microbiol 2011;49: 790–6.

61. Huang B, Troese MJ, Ye S, et al. Anaplasma phagocytophilum APH_1387 is expressed throughout bacterial intracellular development and localizes to the pathogen-occupied vacuolar membrane. Infect Immun 2010;78:1864–73.

62. Demma LJ, Holman RC, McQuiston JH, et al. Epidemiology of human ehrlichiosis and anaplasmosis in the United States, 2001-2002. Am J Trop Med Hyg 2005;73:400–9.

63. Esemu SN, Ndip LM, Ndip RN. Ehrlichia species, probable emerging human pathogens in sub-Saharan Africa: environmental exacerbation. Rev Environ Health 2011;26:269–79.

64. Hidalgo M, Vesga JF, Lizarazo D, et al. A survey of antibodies against Rickettsia rickettsii and Ehrlichia chaffeensis in domestic animals from a rural area of Colombia. Am J Trop Med Hyg 2009;80:1029–30.

65. Marshall GS, Jacobs RF, Schutze GE, et al. Ehrlichia chaffeensis seroprevalence among children in the southeast and south-central regions of the United States. Arch Pediatr Adolesc Med 2002;156:166–70.

66. Bakken JS, Dumler JS, Chen SM, et al. Human granulocytic ehrlichiosis in the upper Midwest United States. A new species emerging? [comment]. JAMA 1994;272:212–8.

67. Walker DH, Paddock CD, Dumler JS. Emerging and re-emerging tick-transmitted rickettsial and ehrlichial infections. Med Clin North Am 2008;92:1345–61.
68. Dong J, Olano JP, McBride JW, et al. Emerging pathogens: challenges and successes of molecular diagnostics. J Mol Diagn 2008;10:185–97.
69. Olano JP, Masters E, Hogrefe W, et al. Human monocytotropic ehrlichiosis, Missouri. Emerg Infect Dis 2003;9:1579–86.
70. Bakken JS, Goellner P, Van Etten M, et al. Seroprevalence of human granulocytic ehrlichiosis among permanent residents of northwestern Wisconsin. Clin Infect Dis 1998;27:1491–6.
71. Nadelman RB, Horowitz HW, Hsieh TC, et al. Simultaneous human granulocytic ehrlichiosis and Lyme borreliosis [comment]. N Engl J Med 1997;337:27–30.
72. Chapman AS, Bakken JS, Folk SM, et al. Diagnosis and management of tick-borne rickettsial diseases: Rocky Mountain spotted fever, ehrlichioses, and anaplasmosis–United States: a practical guide for physicians and other health-care and public health professionals. MMWR Recomm Rep 2006;55:1–27.
73. Buller RS, Arens M, Hmiel SP, et al. Ehrlichia ewingii, a newly recognized agent of human ehrlichiosis. N Engl J Med 1999;341:148–55.
74. Paddock CD, Folk SM, Shore GM, et al. Infections with Ehrlichia chaffeensis and Ehrlichia ewingii in persons coinfected with human immunodeficiency virus. Clin Infect Dis 2001;33:1586–94.
75. Di Sabatino A, Pickard KM, Gordon JN, et al. Evidence for the role of interferon-alfa production by dendritic cells in the Th1 response in celiac disease. Gastroenterology 2007;133:1175–87.
76. Mixson TR, Campbell SR, Gill JS, et al. Prevalence of Ehrlichia, Borrelia, and Rickettsial agents in Amblyomma americanum (Acari: Ixodidae) collected from nine states. J Med Entomol 2006;43:1261–8.
77. Choi KS, Scorpio DG, Barat NC. Msp2 variation in Anaplasma phagocytophilum in vivo does not stimulate T cell immune responses or interferon-gamma production. FEMS Immunol Med Microbiol 2007;49:374–86.
78. Galvao MA, Dumler JS, Mafra CL, et al. Fatal spotted fever rickettsiosis, Minas Gerais, Brazil. Emerg Infect Dis 2003;9:1402–5.
79. Schutze GE, Buckingham SC, Marshall GS, et al. Human monocytic ehrlichiosis in children. Pediatr Infect Dis J 2007;26:475–9.
80. Fichtenbaum CJ, Peterson LR, Weil GJ. Ehrlichiosis presenting as a life-threatening illness with features of the toxic shock syndrome. Am J Med 1993;95:351–7.
81. Hongo I, Bloch KC. Ehrlichia infection of the central nervous system. Curr Treat Options Neurol 2006;8:179–84.
82. Ratnasamy N, Everett ED, Roland WE, et al. Central nervous system manifestations of human ehrlichiosis. Clin Infect Dis 1996;23:314–9.
83. Ismail N, Walker DH, Ghose P, et al. Immune mediators of protective and pathogenic immune responses in patients with mild and fatal human monocytotropic ehrlichiosis. BMC Immunol 2012;13:26.
84. Martin ME, Bunnell JE, Dumler JS. Pathology, immunohistology, and cytokine responses in early phases of human granulocytic ehrlichiosis in a murine model. J Infect Dis 2000;181:374–8.
85. Schutze GE. Ehrlichiosis. Pediatr Infect Dis J 2006;25:71–2.
86. Berry DS, Miller ES, Hooke JA, et al. Ehrlichial meningitis with cerebrospinal fluid morulae. Pediatr Infect Dis J 1999;18:552–5.
87. Arraga-Alvarado C. Human ehrlichiosis [review]. Invest Clin 1994;35:209–22.

88. Horowitz HW, Marks SJ, Weintraub M, et al. Brachial plexopathy associated with human granulocytic ehrlichiosis. Neurology 1996;46:1026–9.

89. Akkoyunlu M, Fikrig E. Gamma interferon dominates the murine cytokine response to the agent of human granulocytic ehrlichiosis and helps to control the degree of early rickettsemia. Infect Immun 2000;68:1827–33.

90. Dunphy PS, Luo T, McBride JW. Ehrlichia moonlighting effectors and interkingdom interactions with the mononuclear phagocyte. Microbes Infect 2013;15: 1005–16.

91. Nandi B, Chatterjee M, Hogle K, et al. Antigen display, T-cell activation, and immune evasion during acute and chronic ehrlichiosis. Infect Immun 2009;77: 4643–53.

92. McBride JW, Walker DH. Progress and obstacles in vaccine development for the ehrlichioses. Expert Rev Vaccines 2010;9:1071–82.

93. Rikihisa Y. Ehrlichia subversion of host innate responses. Curr Opin Microbiol 2006;9:95–101.

94. Lina TT, Dunphy PS, Luo T, et al. Ehrlichia chaffeensis TRP120 activates canonical notch signaling to downregulate TLR2/4 expression and promote intracellular survival. MBio 2016;7(4):e00672–16.

95. Zhu B, Kuriakose JA, Luo T, et al. Ehrlichia chaffeensis TRP120 binds a G+C-rich motif in host cell DNA and exhibits eukaryotic transcriptional activator function. Infect Immun 2011;79:4370–81.

96. Mohan Kumar D, Lin M, Xiong Q, et al. EtpE binding to DNase X induces ehrlichial entry via CD147 and hnRNP-K recruitment, followed by mobilization of N-WASP and actin. MBio 2015;6. e01541-15.

97. Mohan Kumar D, Yamaguchi M, Miura K, et al. Ehrlichia chaffeensis uses its surface protein EtpE to bind GPI-anchored protein DNase X and trigger entry into mammalian cells. PLoS Pathog 2013;9:e1003666.

98. Lin M, Liu H, Xiong Q, et al. Ehrlichia secretes Etf-1 to induce autophagy and capture nutrients for its growth through RAB5 and class III phosphatidylinositol 3-kinase. Autophagy 2016;12:2145–66.

99. Rikihisa Y. Mechanisms of obligatory intracellular infection with Anaplasma phagocytophilum. Clin Microbiol Rev 2011;24:469–89.

100. Cheng Z, Lin M, Rikihisa Y. Ehrlichia chaffeensis proliferation begins with NtrY/NtrX and PutA/GlnA upregulation and CtrA degradation induced by proline and glutamine uptake. MBio 2014;5:e02141.

101. Rikihisa Y. Molecular pathogenesis of ehrlichia chaffeensis infection. Annu Rev Microbiol 2015;69:283–304.

102. Lee EH, Rikihisa Y. Protein kinase A-mediated inhibition of gamma interferon-induced tyrosine phosphorylation of Janus kinases and latent cytoplasmic transcription factors in human monocytes by Ehrlichia chaffeensis. Infect Immun 1998;66:2514–20.

103. Barnewall RE, Ohashi N, Rikihisa Y. Ehrlichia chaffeensis and E. sennetsu, but not the human granulocytic ehrlichiosis agent, colocalize with transferrin receptor and up-regulate transferrin receptor mRNA by activating iron-responsive protein 1. Infect Immun 1999;67:2258–65.

104. Cahir-McFarland ED, Davidson DM, Schauer SL, et al. NF-kappa B inhibition causes spontaneous apoptosis in Epstein-Barr virus-transformed lymphoblastoid cells. Proc Natl Acad Sci U S A 2000;97:6055–60.

105. Chattoraj P, Yang Q, Khandai A, et al. TLR2 and Nod2 mediate resistance or susceptibility to fatal intracellular Ehrlichia infection in murine models of ehrlichiosis. PLoS One 2013;8:e58514.

106. MacNamara KC, Jones M, Martin O, et al. Transient activation of hematopoietic stem and progenitor cells by IFNgamma during acute bacterial infection. PLoS One 2011;6:e28669.

107. MacNamara KC, Racine R, Chatterjee M, et al. Diminished hematopoietic activity associated with alterations in innate and adaptive immunity in a mouse model of human monocytic ehrlichiosis. Infect Immun 2009;77:4061–9.

108. Dierberg KL, Dumler JS. Lymph node hemophagocytosis in rickettsial diseases: a pathogenetic role for CD8 T lymphocytes in human monocytic ehrlichiosis (HME)? BMC Infect Dis 2006;6:121.

109. Hamburg BJ, Storch GA, Micek ST, et al. The importance of early treatment with doxycycline in human ehrlichiosis. Medicine (Baltimore) 2008;87:53–60.

110. Kumar N, Goyal J, Goel A, et al. Macrophage activation syndrome secondary to human monocytic ehrlichiosis. Indian J Hematol Blood Transfus 2014;30:145–7.

111. Thomas LD, Hongo I, Bloch KC, et al. Human ehrlichiosis in transplant recipients. Am J Transplant 2007;7:1641–7.

112. Brady RC, Bissler JJ. Renal, hepatic, and marrow dysfunction in a patient with chronic renal insufficiency. Pediatr Nephrol 2003;18:293–6.

113. Sehdev AE, Dumler JS. Hepatic pathology in human monocytic ehrlichiosis. Ehrlichia chaffeensis infection. Am J Clin Pathol 2003;119:859–65.

114. de Sousa R, Ismail N, Doria-Nobrega S, et al. The presence of eschars, but not greater severity, in Portuguese patients infected with Israeli spotted fever. Ann N Y Acad Sci 2005;1063:197–202.

115. Ismail N, Stevenson HL, Walker DH. Role of tumor necrosis factor alpha (TNF-alpha) and interleukin-10 in the pathogenesis of severe murine monocytotropic ehrlichiosis: increased resistance of TNF receptor p55- and p75-deficient mice to fatal ehrlichial infection. Infect Immun 2006;74:1846–56.

116. Thirumalapura NR, Stevenson HL, Walker DH, et al. Protective heterologous immunity against fatal ehrlichiosis and lack of protection following homologous challenge. Infect Immun 2008;76:1920–30.

117. Ismail N, Crossley EC, Stevenson HL, et al. Relative importance of T-cell subsets in monocytotropic ehrlichiosis: a novel effector mechanism involved in Ehrlichia-induced immunopathology in murine ehrlichiosis. Infect Immun 2007;75: 4608–20.

118. Walker DH, Dumler JS. The role of CD8 T lymphocytes in rickettsial infections. Semin Immunopathol 2015;37:289–99.

119. Ghose P, Ali AQ, Fang R, et al. The interaction between IL-18 and IL-18 receptor limits the magnitude of protective immunity and enhances pathogenic responses following infection with intracellular bacteria. J Immunol 2011;187: 1333–46.

120. Yang Q, Stevenson HL, Scott MJ, et al. Type I interferon contributes to noncanonical inflammasome activation, mediates immunopathology, and impairs protective immunity during fatal infection with lipopolysaccharide-negative ehrlichiae. Am J Pathol 2014;185(2):446–61.

121. Deretic V, Saitoh T, Akira S. Autophagy in infection, inflammation and immunity. Nat Rev Immunol 2013;13:722–37.

122. Kanneganti TD. Central roles of NLRs and inflammasomes in viral infection. Nat Rev Immunol 2010;10:688–98.

123. Aachoui Y, Leaf IA, Hagar JA, et al. Caspase-11 protects against bacteria that escape the vacuole. Science 2013;339:975–8.

124. Antonopoulos C, Russo HM, El Sanadi C, et al. Caspase-8 as an effector and regulator of NLRP3 inflammasome signaling. J Biol Chem 2015;290:20167–84.

125. Broz P, Monack DM. Measuring inflammasome activation in response to bacterial infection. Methods Mol Biol 2013;1040:65–84.
126. Mattner J, Debord KL, Ismail N, et al. Exogenous and endogenous glycolipid antigens activate NKT cells during microbial infections. Nature 2005;434:525–9.
127. Stevenson HL, Estes MD, Thirumalapura NR, et al. Natural killer cells promote tissue injury and systemic inflammatory responses during fatal Ehrlichia-induced toxic shock-like syndrome. Am J Pathol 2010;177:766–76.
128. Stevenson HL, Crossley EC, Thirumalapura N, et al. Regulatory roles of CD1d-restricted NKT cells in the induction of toxic shock-like syndrome in an animal model of fatal ehrlichiosis. Infect Immun 2008;76:1434–44.
129. Chan WK, Rujkijyanont P, Neale G, et al. Multiplex and genome-wide analyses reveal distinctive properties of KIR+ and CD56+ T cells in human blood. J Immunol 2013;191:1625–36.
130. Reneer DV, Troese MJ, Huang B, et al. Anaplasma phagocytophilum PSGL-1-independent infection does not require Syk and leads to less efficient AnkA delivery. Cell Microbiol 2008;10:1827–38.
131. Ge Y, Yoshiie K, Kuribayashi F, et al. Anaplasma phagocytophilum inhibits human neutrophil apoptosis via upregulation of bfl-1, maintenance of mitochondrial membrane potential and prevention of caspase 3 activation. Cell Microbiol 2005;7:29–38.
132. Troese MJ, Carlyon JA. Anaplasma phagocytophilum dense-cored organisms mediate cellular adherence through recognition of human P-selectin glycoprotein ligand 1. Infect Immun 2009;77:4018–27.
133. Troese MJ, Kahlon A, Ragland SA, et al. Proteomic analysis of Anaplasma phagocytophilum during infection of human myeloid cells identifies a protein that is pronouncedly upregulated on the infectious dense-cored cell. Infect Immun 2011;79:4696–707.
134. Choi KS, Scorpio DG, Dumler JS. Anaplasma phagocytophilum ligation to toll-like receptor (TLR) 2, but not to TLR4, activates macrophages for nuclear factor-kappa B nuclear translocation. J Infect Dis 2004;189:1921–5.
135. Cheng Z, Miura K, Popov VL, et al. Insights into the CtrA regulon in development of stress resistance in obligatory intracellular pathogen Ehrlichia chaffeensis. Mol Microbiol 2011;82:1217–34.
136. Wang X, Shaw DK, Hammond HL, et al. The prostaglandin E2-EP3 receptor Axis regulates Anaplasma phagocytophilum-mediated NLRC4 inflammasome activation. PLoS Pathog 2016;12:e1005803.
137. Bouwman LI, de Zoete MR, Bleumink-Pluym NM, et al. Inflammasome activation by Campylobacter jejuni. J Immunol 2014;193:4548–57.
138. Case CL, Kohler LJ, Lima JB, et al. Caspase-11 stimulates rapid flagellin-independent pyroptosis in response to Legionella pneumophila. Proc Natl Acad Sci U S A 2013;110:1851–6.
139. Koebel C, Kern A, Edouard S, et al. Human granulocytic anaplasmosis in eastern France: clinical presentation and laboratory diagnosis. Diagn Microbiol Infect Dis 2012;72:214–8.
140. Seidman D, Ojogun N, Walker NJ, et al. Anaplasma phagocytophilum surface protein AipA mediates invasion of mammalian host cells. Cell Microbiol 2014;16:1133–45.
141. Bakken JS, Dumler JS. Human granulocytic anaplasmosis. Infect Dis Clin North Am 2015;29:341–55.
142. Dumler JS, Barat NC, Barat CE, et al. Human granulocytic anaplasmosis and macrophage activation. Clin Infect Dis 2007;45:199–204.

143. Assi MA, Yao JD, Walker RC. Lyme disease followed by human granulocytic anaplasmosis in a kidney transplant recipient. Transpl Infect Dis 2007;9:66–72.
144. Bitsaktsis C, Huntington J, Winslow G. Production of IFN-gamma by CD4 T cells is essential for resolving ehrlichia infection. J Immunol 2004;172:6894–901.
145. Bitsaktsis C, Winslow G. Fatal recall responses mediated by CD8 T cells during intracellular bacterial challenge infection. J Immunol 2006;177:4644–51.
146. Kim HY, Rikihisa Y. Roles of p38 mitogen-activated protein kinase, NF-kappaB, and protein kinase C in proinflammatory cytokine mRNA expression by human peripheral blood leukocytes, monocytes, and neutrophils in response to Anaplasma phagocytophila. Infect Immun 2002;70:4132–41.
147. Winslow GM, Bitsaktsis C, Yager E. Susceptibility and resistance to monocytic ehrlichiosis in the mouse. Ann N Y Acad Sci 2005;1063:395–402.
148. Olano JP, Walker DH. Human ehrlichioses. Med Clin North Am 2002;86:375–92.
149. Lee EH, Rikihisa Y. Anti-Ehrlichia chaffeensis antibody complexed with E. chaffeensis induces potent proinflammatory cytokine mRNA expression in human monocytes through sustained reduction of IkappaB-alpha and activation of NF-kappaB. Infect Immun 1997;65:2890–7.
150. Bitsaktsis C, Nandi B, Racine R, et al. T-Cell-independent humoral immunity is sufficient for protection against fatal intracellular ehrlichia infection. Infect Immun 2007;75:4933–41.
151. Li JS, Chu F, Reilly A, et al. Antibodies highly effective in SCID mice during infection by the intracellular bacterium Ehrlichia chaffeensis are of picomolar affinity and exhibit preferential epitope and isotype utilization. J Immunol 2002;169:1419–25.
152. Racine R, Chatterjee M, Winslow GM. CD11c expression identifies a population of extrafollicular antigen-specific splenic plasmablasts responsible for CD4 T-independent antibody responses during intracellular bacterial infection. J Immunol 2008;181:1375–85.
153. Racine R, Jones DD, Chatterjee M, et al. Impaired germinal center responses and suppression of local IgG production during intracellular bacterial infection. J Immunol 2010;184:5085–93.
154. Liddell AM, Sumner JW, Paddock CD, et al. Reinfection with Ehrlichia chaffeensis in a liver transplant recipient. Clin Infect Dis 2002;34:1644–7.
155. Bakken JS, Dumler JS. Clinical diagnosis and treatment of human granulocytotropic anaplasmosis. Ann N Y Acad Sci 2006;1078:236–47.
156. Chan K, Marras SA, Parveen N. Sensitive multiplex PCR assay to differentiate Lyme spirochetes and emerging pathogens Anaplasma phagocytophilum and Babesia microti. BMC Microbiol 2013;13:295.
157. Doyle CK, Labruna MB, Breitschwerdt EB, et al. Detection of medically important Ehrlichia by quantitative multicolor TaqMan real-time polymerase chain reaction of the dsb gene. J Mol Diagn 2005;7:504–10.
158. Kocianova E, Kost'anova Z, Stefanidesova K, et al. Serologic evidence of Anaplasma phagocytophilum infections in patients with a history of tick bite in central Slovakia. Wien Klin Wochenschr 2008;120:427–31.
159. Glaser C, Christie L, Bloch KC. Rickettsial and ehrlichial infections. Handb Clin Neurol 2010;96:143–58.
160. Shields K, Cumming M, Rios J, et al. Transfusion-associated Anaplasma phagocytophilum infection in a pregnant patient with thalassemia trait: a case report. Transfusion 2015;55:719–25.
161. Caldwell CW, Everett ED, McDonald G, et al. Lymphocytosis of gamma/delta T cells in human ehrlichiosis. Am J Clin Pathol 1995;103:761–6.

162. Caldwell CW, Everett ED, McDonald G, et al. Apoptosis of gamma/delta T cells in human ehrlichiosis. Am J Clin Pathol 1996;105:640–6.

163. Mayne PJ. Clinical determinants of Lyme borreliosis, babesiosis, bartonellosis, anaplasmosis, and ehrlichiosis in an Australian cohort. Int J Gen Med 2015;8: 15–26.

164. Olano JP, Walker DH. Diagnosing emerging and reemerging infectious diseases: the pivotal role of the pathologist. Arch Pathol Lab Med 2011;135:83–91.

165. Paddock CD, Childs JE. Ehrlichia chaffeensis: a prototypical emerging pathogen. Clin Microbiol Rev 2003;16:37–64.

166. Standaert SM, Yu T, Scott MA, et al. Primary isolation of Ehrlichia chaffeensis from patients with febrile illnesses: clinical and molecular characteristics. J Infect Dis 2000;181:1082–8.

167. Bloch KC, Tang YW, Hillstron L. Predictors of tick-borne rickettsial disease among patients hospitalized with encephalitis. San Francisco (CA): Infectious Diseases Society of America; 2005.

168. Dumler JS. Anaplasma and ehrlichia infection. Ann N Y Acad Sci 2005;1063: 361–73.

169. Wormser GP, Dattwyler RJ, Shapiro ED, et al. The clinical assessment, treatment, and prevention of Lyme disease, human granulocytic anaplasmosis, and babesiosis: clinical practice guidelines by the Infectious Diseases Society of America. Clin Infect Dis 2006;43:1089–134.

Clostridium difficile

Scott R. Curry, MD

KEYWORDS

- *Clostridium difficile* • CDI • Diagnosis • Epidemiology
- Fecal microbiota transplantation • FMT

KEY POINTS

- *C difficile* is widely distributed in nature but concentrated within health care environments.
- Asymptomatic carriage of humans with *C difficile* is common, posing a significant challenge for the laboratory diagnosis of *C difficile* infection (CDI).
- CDI poses a substantial threat to the health of hospitalized patients and other subgroups of immunocompromised patients.
- The collateral protective effect of an individual's microbiome may be as important as host immune defenses for CDI.
- Fecal microbiota transplantation (FMT) is emerging as the most effective treatment of patients with recurrent CDI.

OVERVIEW

Clostridium difficile was identified as the leading cause of antibiotic-associated diarrhea and colitis in 1978, but since 2001 *C difficile* infections (CDIs) have evolved from sporadic complications of antimicrobial therapy to severe, sometimes fatal, events that have become an endemic threat to the health of hospitalized and immunosuppressed patients worldwide. This article discusses the changing epidemiology, clinical and laboratory diagnosis, pathogenesis, and treatment of CDI.

MICROBIOLOGY

C difficile is an obligate anaerobic, spore-forming, gram-positive rod first described in 1935 as *Bacillus difficilis* in the fecal flora of healthy infants.[1] The organism remained unrecognized as a cause of human infection until 1977 when it was identified as the cause of what had previously been referred to as antibiotic-associated colitis.[2,3] Hall and O'Toole's[1] species name reflected difficulty of isolating *C difficile* from other

This article is an update of an article previously published in Clinics in Laboratory Medicine, Volume 30, Issue 1, March 2010.
Disclosure Statement: The author has nothing to disclose.
Division of Infectious Diseases, Medical University of South Carolina, 1215 Rutledge Tower, 135 Rutledge Avenue, MSC 752, Charleston, SC 29425, USA
E-mail address: currysr@musc.edu

anaerobic and facultative stool flora, which was mostly attributable to its slow growth (40–70 minutes doubling time). C difficile is exquisitely aerointolerant during logarithmic growth phases when vegetative cells predominate,[4] making it difficult for laboratories not equipped with anaerobic chambers to passage the organism before sporulation occurs at approximately 48 to 72 hours. Laboratories equipped with anaerobic jar systems are delayed in the ability to isolate the organism because of the need for a minimum 48 hours between passages to avoid fatal oxygen intoxication of fresh cultures.

Culture of C difficile has been unfairly perceived as difficult, however, because selective media have been refined to isolate the organism from fecal and environmental specimens (**Fig. 1**).[5–7] These media capitalize on the organism's intrinsic resistance to cefoxitin and cycloserine and the ability of C difficile to use fructose and mannitol as carbohydrate sources; Stickland reactions play a central role in the organism's biosynthetic pathways and account for the organism's alkalization of undefined peptone-based media, which are widely used with neutral red to indicate C difficile growth in liquid and agar media (see **Fig. 1**), usually within 48 hours of incubation.[8] Sodium taurocholate, a bile salt, has been shown to be vital to the germination of C difficile endospores and is an essential component in selective media.[9,10]

Once isolated, C difficile is readily subcultured to nonselective media, such as 5% sheep blood agar on which it assumes its characteristic irregular ground-glass colonial

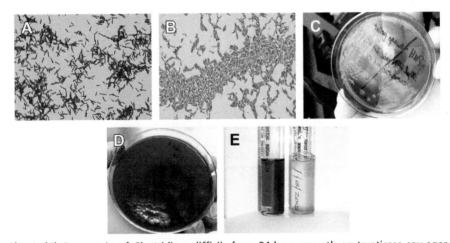

Fig. 1. (A) Gram stain of *Clostridium difficile* from 24-hour growth on trypticase soy agar with 5% sheep blood. The vegetative cell bodies are often gram-negative during early growth; note the abundant subterminal endospores that do not swell the parent cell (original magnification ×100). (B) Malachite green stain of 48-hour growth of C difficile. The safranin counterstain renders vegetative cells pink, whereas the endospores stain green, revealing their ovoid shape (original magnification ×100). (C) A 48-hour growth of C difficile on typical selective agar medium, C difficile basal agar with moxalactam and norfloxacin, which uses norfloxacin and moxalactam as selective antibiotics to allow primary isolation from stool specimens. Other media use combinations of cycloserine and cefoxitin as selective antibiotics (cycloserine cefoxitin fructose agar). Neutral red is turned *yellow* by C difficile growth. (D) Typical appearance of C difficile colonies on trypticase soy agar with 5% sheep blood at 48 hours. Colonies are nonhemolytic. (E) A selective broth medium for isolation of C difficile, cycloserine cefoxitin mannitol broth with taurocholate, and lysozyme. The tube at *right* shows turbidity and growth of C difficile at 24 hours, with obvious alkalinization of the neutral red indicator. The tube at *left* is a negative control.

morphology without hemolysis (**Fig. 2**). Although *C difficile* colonies vary greatly in size (more motile strains have maximum colony widths of 12–15 mm), they fluoresce under UV illumination and exhibit a characteristic odor often referred to as "horse dung" or "barn" odor. This phenotypic feature results from the ability of the organism to ferment tyrosine into *p*-cresol, a phenolic compound for which the species has considerable tolerance and which can be used to distinguish the organism from other clostridia using high-performance liquid chromatography.[11,12] Smaller colonies of *C difficile* are difficult to distinguish morphologically from those of other nonhemolytic *Clostridium* spp, but rapid biochemical confirmation with L-proline aminopeptidase spot disk activity can provide confirmation of suspected *C difficile*.[13]

Chromogenic commercial media have also been developed that allow for more rapid isolation of *C difficile* (usually as colorless or grey-black colonies on a blue background within 24 hours), but these media often allow for growth of non-*difficile* clostridia.[14] Matrix-assisted laser desorption/ionization time-of-flight mass spectrometer platforms are readily able to distinguish *C difficile* from other clostridia in these circumstances.[14–16]

Culture of *C difficile* is primarily a research tool used in the evaluation of diagnostic tests and to recover isolates for outbreak investigation and molecular epidemiology. *C difficile* isolates are maintained nearly indefinitely at room temperature as spore stocks or as vegetative cells in chopped meat medium, although many laboratories are in the

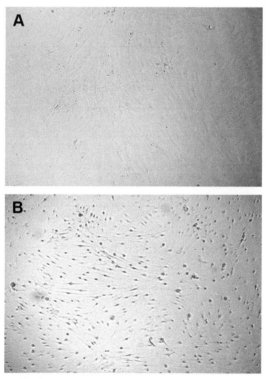

Fig. 2. (*A*) Negative cell culture cytotoxicity assay. Human fibroblasts remain spindle-shaped and in contact with each other. (*B*) Positive cell culture cytotoxicity assay revealing cytopathic effects of *C difficile* toxin B causing cell rounding and separation. (*Courtesy of* Ray Hariri, PhD, Pittsburgh, PA, USA.)

habit of storing the organism in frozen glycerol stocks.[17,18] Because nontoxigenic strains of *C difficile* are commonplace, culture of the organism for clinical purposes must be followed by confirmation of toxin production. This is done either using molecular tests for the presence of toxin genes or by performing cytotoxicity assays or enzyme immunoassays (EIAs) on cell-free culture supernatants (discussed in section on pathogenesis and diagnosis). For phenotypic toxin testing, use of complex media without glucose, fructose, and mannitol (present in most of the primarily selective media for the organism) may be important to minimize the effect of rapidly metabolized carbon sources in repression of toxin synthesis.[19] The glucosyltransferase activities of toxins A and B in *C difficile* have been used to devise selective media that can identify toxigenic strains in a single step using the presence of an insoluble blue product around colonies of toxigenic strains at 48 hours of incubation, but to date this methodology has not undergone a wide-scale validation and may miss some strains expressing toxin at low levels.[20]

MOLECULAR EPIDEMIOLOGY AND STRAIN TYPING

For the purposes of tracking global and local molecular epidemiology of *C difficile*, several strain typing systems have been devised (**Table 1**). For tracking global linages, pulsed field gel electrophoresis (PFGE) is the method generally preferred by the US Centers for Disease Control and Prevention,[21,22] whereas European centers and others have preferred polymerase chain reaction (PCR) ribotyping.[23] Both methods are band-based and require sets of reference isolates and suffer from a degree of

Table 1
Laboratory typing methods for CDI

Method	High-Throughput	Portable	Determines Lineage	Discriminatory Capacity	Authors, References
Toxinotyping	No	Yes	No	Low	Rupnik et al,[188] 1998
Pulsed field gel electrophoresis	No	No	Yes	Low-moderate	Corkill et al,[22] 2000
Restriction endonuclease analysis	No	No	Yes	Moderate-high	Clabots et al,[27] 1993
Polymerase chain reaction ribotyping	Yes	No	Yes	Low-moderate	Stubbs et al,[23] 1999
Multilocus sequence typing	Yes	Yes	Yes	Low	Griffiths et al,[24] 2010; Lemee et al,[189] 2004
tcdC genotyping	Yes	Yes	Yes	Low	Curry et al,[25] 2007; Dingle et al,[26] 2011
Multiple locus variable number of tandem repeats analysis	Yes	Yes	No	High	Marsh et al,[29] 2006; van den Berg et al,[30] 2007
Whole genome sequencing	No	Yes	Yes	High	Eyre et al,[28] 2013; Didelot et al,[190] 2012

subjectivity, but both methods are able to separate *C difficile* lineages that correspond to a large degree with the 380 lineages of *C difficile* identified using a more objective and technically demanding method based on Sanger sequencing of *C difficile* house-keeping genes, multilocus sequence typing (MLST).[24] A single locus typing scheme based on sequencing of the *tcdC* gene has been devised and can serve to distinguish the lineages of toxigenic strains, but this scheme is not suited for typing of nontoxigenic strains.[25,26] MLST and *tcdC* typing are both entirely portable, with a public database of sequence types maintained by the University of Oxford (http://pubmlst.org/cdifficile). PFGE, ribotyping, MLST, and *tcdC* genotyping are insufficiently discriminatory for source attributions or tracking hospital outbreaks, for which restriction endonuclease analysis, multilocus variable number of tandem repeats analysis, and whole genome sequencing are more suited, each representing progressively increased discriminatory capacity.[27–30] There has been considerable enthusiasm for adoption of whole genome sequencing–based methods, but the high cost and lack of a standardized analysis scheme for whole genome sequencing data are barriers to the wide-scale adoption of this method.

ECOLOGY, HOST RANGE, AND DISTRIBUTION

C difficile is ubiquitous and widely distributed in nature (**Table 2**).[31] It is found easily in soil and sewage and has been found in the feces of most mammals.[31] *C difficile* has occasionally been described as a veterinary pathogen, particularly in piglets, calves, and some avian species,[32,33] but its epidemiology in animals is not nearly as well-described as it is for *Clostridium perfringens* in animal husbandry. The original animal model for CDI was the Syrian hamster, which suffers a lethal colitis after antibiotic preexposure.[34] More recently, mouse models of CDI have been developed that more closely parallel nonlethal CDI in humans, including the development of relapsed infection after recovery.[35] To date, however, there is scant evidence that CDI occurs in nature in the absence of antimicrobial use.

Despite initial concern that *C difficile* is widespread in the food supply, most prevalence studies suggest that the prevalence of *C difficile* is low and occurs at low colony counts (**Table 3**).[36,37] *C difficile* strain typing has suggested that some high initial

Table 2		
Prevalence of toxigenic *Clostridium difficile* from sampling of various sources in South Wales		
Source	N	Toxigenic *Clostridium difficile* (%)
Domestic animals	200	3 (1.5)
Farm animals	524	4 (0.8)
Fish	107	0
Soil	104	9 (8.6)
Hospitals	380	72 (18.9)
Nursing homes	275	4 (1.5)
Houses	350	3 (0.9)
Dorms	200	3 (1.5)
Water	110	36 (32.7)
Vegetables	300	5 (1.7)
Total	2580	140 (5.4)

Adapted from al Saif N, Brazier JS. The distribution of *Clostridium difficile* in the environment of South Wales. J Med Microbiol 1996;45(2):135.

Table 3
Prevalence of *Clostridium difficile* in the human food supply

Prevalence (%)	95% Confidence Interval	Region	Product Sampled	Authors, References
37/88 (42.0)	31.6–53.1	Tucson, AZ	Ground meat	Songer et al,[191] 2009
8/500 (1.6)	0.69–3.1	Netherlands	Retail meats	de Boer et al,[192] 2011
5/111 (4.5)	1.5–10.2	Ontario, CA	Vegetables	Metcalf et al,[193] 2010
0/46 (0)	0–7.7	Switzerland	Ground beef	Hoffer et al,[194] 2010
26/203 (12.8)	8.5–18.2	Ontario, CA	Retail chicken	Weese et al,[195] 2010
3/100 (3)	0.6–8.5	Switzerland	Ground meat	Jobstl et al,[196] 2010
3/50 (6)	1.3–16.6	Pennsylvania	Ground veal	Houser et al,[197] 2012
2/82 (2.4)	0.3–8.5	Sweden	Ground meat	Von Abercron et al,[198] 2009
4/32 (12.5)	3.5–29.0	Texas	Poultry meat	Harvey et al,[199] 2011
3/40 (7.5)	1.6–20.4	Texas	Ground meat	Harvey et al,[200] 2011
2/102 (2.0)	2.4–6.9	Pennsylvania	Ground meat	Curry et al,[36] 2012

prevalence estimates of *C difficile* in meat products may have arisen from laboratory contamination events, and thus far there is no direct evidence that *C difficile* is a food-borne illness.[38,39] In contrast, environmental studies have consistently identified health care environments, including outpatient clinics, as heavily contaminated with *C difficile*.[6,40,41]

DISINFECTION, SURVIVAL, AND LABORATORY INFECTION

The endospores of *C difficile* are resistant to heat, 70% ethanol used in hand sanitizers, and the quaternary ammonium detergents used as hospital and laboratory disinfectants, but sodium hypochlorite-based solutions are capable of inactivating spores.[42] *C difficile* spores are known to have nearly indefinite viability, demonstrating only $0.5\log_{10}$ reduction in viability after 14 months of storage on steel disks at room temperature.[18] The viability of *C difficile* spores contaminating hospital environments also declines over time, but not at a rate that is below the infectious inoculum ($ID_{50} = 5$ spores/cm^2) in the mouse model of CDI.[41,43] Sodium hypochlorite (chlorine bleach) at a concentration of 5000 ppm (achieved with 10% aqueous solution of standard household bleach in distilled, deionized water) at 10 minutes of contact time results in a 6 $\log_{10}$ ($\geq$99.9999%) reduction in the viability of *C difficile* spores, although lesser concentrations of bleach take up to 30 minutes for the same level of activity.[44]

Occupancy of a room previously occupied by patients known to have CDI and by patients previously receiving antimicrobials has been identified as a significant risk for development of CDI among subsequent hospital room occupants, highlighting the need to provide adequate terminal disinfection to prevent transmission to new patients.[45,46] Previous studies have reported adoption of sodium hypochlorite cleaning of hospital environments as key elements in the control of CDI epidemics in hospitals,[47] but more recently less caustic alternative agents, such as combinations of hydrogen peroxide and peracetic acid, have been developed as terminal disinfectants.[48] The development of fully automated ultraviolet irradiation devices and hydrogen peroxide vapor systems for disinfection of hospital rooms holds promise as a means to enhance the effectiveness of hospital disinfection, but these devices do not eliminate the need to perform routine cleaning of the organic soil burden on hospital surfaces and add 30 to 60 minutes to the process of cleaning a hospital room, increasing considerably the cost of this approach.[49,50] Nonetheless, centers that have adopted these systems have observed significant decreases in health care–associated CDI rates.[51–53]

Laboratory-acquired CDI has been anecdotally reported. Both reported cases involved young women who were working with *C difficile* on open benches and using alcohol (which is inactive against *C difficile* spores) to disinfect laboratory work surfaces.[54] Only one of the two cases had known antibiotic exposures, although the case in which no antibiotic exposure was noted was self-limited and resolved without treatment.[54] Nonetheless, Bouza and colleagues[54] recommended that all laboratory work with *C difficile* take place in biologic safety cabinets using appropriate barrier precautions and appropriate terminal disinfectants active against *C difficile* spores.

ASYMPTOMATIC CARRIAGE OF *CLOSTRIDIUM DIFFICILE*

Healthy, nonhospitalized ambulatory adults are commonly colonized with *C difficile*, and the colonization of 5% to 15% of adults is often transient.[55–57] A prospective survey found that 26% of 428 hospitalized patients in a medical ward acquired *C difficile*. In this study, only 38% developed symptoms consistent with CDI by 11 months, indicating that 62% of patients who acquired *C difficile* were asymptomatically colonized.[58] In a later study by Clabots and colleagues,[59] 21% of all admissions to a single medical ward at a Veterans Affairs hospital were positive for *C difficile* carriage during a 9-month period. Of these, 86% were asymptomatic carriers. The predominant mode of acquisition in this study was hospital-associated in 41% of admissions. Molecular typing of recovered isolates revealed 19 instances of within-hospital transmission among asymptomatic patients. Acquisition of the same strains was documented within the same hospital room separated in time by up to 24 weeks, suggesting that environmental contamination contributes to *C difficile* transmission. The study also documented transmission between pairs of patients who were in rooms far separated from each other, suggesting transmission of *C difficile* spores on the hands of health care workers to new ward admissions.[59]

Subsequent mathematical models of CDI have suggested that transmission within hospitals solely from symptomatic *C difficile* patients is inadequate to account for sustained endemic transmission within hospitals; the contribution of asymptomatic carriers was estimated to be particularly significant if transmission from these carriers was common.[60]

The contribution of asymptomatic carriers to incident CDI has been further estimated in recent studies. Eyre and colleagues[28] performed a population-based study of 1250 CDI cases occurring 2007 to 2011 in Oxfordshire, United Kingdom. Using whole genome sequencing of *C difficile* isolates, they showed that 45% of all incident CDI cases were genetically distinct from all previous cases diagnosed in the region, suggesting that sources beyond symptomatic patients were important in CDI transmission. Using multilocus variable number of tandem repeats analysis genotyping of incident CDI and a concurrent cohort of individuals colonized with *C difficile* at a single medical center in Pittsburgh, Pennsylvania during a 119-day period, Curry and colleagues[61] determined that 17 of 56 (30%) and 16 of 56 (29%) of incident CDI cases could be traced to other symptomatic CDI patients and *C difficile* carriers, respectively. In a 15-month prospective study (of inpatients) in six Canadian hospitals, 117 of 4143 (2.8%) and 123 of 4143 (3.0%) had health care–associated CDI and colonization, respectively, although direct links between these cohorts was not established by strain typing.[62] Longtin and colleagues[63] performed a controlled intervention study to examine the effect of screening incoming admissions to a single Canadian hospital for *C difficile* colonization from 2013 to 2015, demonstrating that simple contact isolation measures for the 4.8% of admissions identified as carriers of *C difficile* resulted in an observed rate of hospital-acquired CDI of 3.0 infections per 10,000 patient-days compared with 6.9 infections per 10,000 patient-days in the preintervention period. Vertical controls based on active surveillance for *C difficile* within health care facilities hold promise as a means to control CDI.

CLINICAL PRESENTATION AND PROGNOSIS

Asymptomatic carriers are by far the most prevalent group among those individuals who are culture-positive for toxin-producing *C difficile*, representing 62% to 86% of hospitalized individuals with *C difficile*–positive stools in previous prospective studies.[58,59] For the minority who develop CDI, the infection exists on a continuum from mild diarrhea to fulminant colitis. Few descriptive series of CDI have been published, but in the pre-2001 era, development of semi-formed diarrhea more than 7 days after antimicrobial exposure was the most common presentation among a series of 43 inpatients.[64] Leukocytosis is a common feature of CDI, which has been found to be the most common cause for unexplained leukocytosis among inpatients and the fourth most common cause for leukocytosis overall.[65,66] Fever is seen in only 50% of cases, and bloody diarrhea is seen in a distinct minority of cases.[64] Rapid increases in leukocytosis, abdominal distention or pain, and sudden cessation of diarrhea are poor prognostic signs that have been anecdotally reported in cases of fulminant colitis.[67]

Several severity score indices for CDI have been developed to best predict CDI patients at risk for death, colectomy, or intensive care unit admission attributable to CDI; fever, leukocytosis, hypoalbuminemia, and abdominal distension were independent predictors of severe CDI in one early study.[68] Subsequent multicenter cohort studies have suggested that a three-point scale based on age greater than or equal to 65 years, peak serum creatinine greater than or equal to 2 mg/dL, and peak peripheral blood leukocyte count greater than or equal to 20,000 cells/µL can be used to predict approximately 75% of patients at risk for severe CDI.[69] A subsequent prospective cohort has resulted in a bedside scoring system based on age, treatment with systemic antibiotics, leukocyte count, albumin, and serum creatinine (ATLAS score 0–10) to predict cure among patients with CDI,[70] and similar prediction rules for recurrence have also been developed.[71] The clinical utility of these scores in management of CDI, an infection characterized by occasionally abrupt changes in clinical severity, is not yet established.

The incubation period for CDI remains unknown, particularly because the incubation period can be defined either from the time of first exposure to the organism, from the first exposure to antibiotics, or from the first appearance of organism in stools until the onset of symptoms. In studies of healthy volunteers without diarrhea, oral administration of nontoxigenic *C difficile* spores results in fecal shedding within 2 to 4 days,[72] but this may not reflect the dynamics of fecal shedding in hospitalized patients. Early studies of hospitalized patients suggested that CDI probably occurred within 7 days of the first appearance of *C difficile* in stool,[73] and beyond this several inpatient cohort studies suggested that patients who did not manifest symptoms of CDI by 7 days of appearance in stool were at reduced risk of subsequent CDI compared with noncolonized patients in the same cohorts.[74] Observational evidence indicates that patients remain at risk for CDI for up to 12 weeks after exposure to antimicrobials, however,[75,76] with the onset of CDI occurring up to 60 days (median, 20.3 days) from the time of hospital discharge.[77] The discrepancies in these observations regarding the potential incubation period for CDI may reflect that follow-up in the initial hospital cohort studies was limited to hospital discharge, and the cohorts were small and may not have included large numbers of severely immunosuppressed patients at high risk for CDI.

EPIDEMIOLOGY OF *CLOSTRIDIUM DIFFICILE* INFECTION

Age greater than or equal to 65, exposure to antimicrobials, and length of stay in a health care facility have all been independently associated with risk for CDI.[78] In addition, age greater than 65 years has been repeatedly associated with an increased risk of symptomatic infection.[79,80] CDI epidemiology changed dramatically after 2000, with an increase in disease incidence and severity, including fulminant colitis, colectomy, and death described at several large hospitals worldwide.[21,81,82] In the United States, *C difficile* incidence doubled from 1996 to 2003.[79] A newly emergent epidemic strain of *C difficile*, which was rarely encountered before 2000 and that became the most prevalent strain causing 30% to 50% of CDI cases, was associated with this phenomenon.[21,81] The epidemic strain has been named NAP1 by PFGE, 027 by PCR ribotyping, BI by restriction endonuclease analysis typing, and ST1 by MLST/*tcdC* genotyping and is usually referred to as NAP1/BI/027.[83]

The causal association of the emergence of this epidemic lineage of *C difficile* and severe CDI is uncertain. In a large population-based surveillance study of 2057 CDI cases with available stain typing data, severe outcomes and death occurred in 4.9% and 2.7% of cases, respectively, and NAP1 strains (28.4% of cases) were associated with severe outcomes and death after adjusting for other confounding risks with adjusted odds ratios of 1.66 and 2.12, respectively.[84] A European study noted that ribotype 078 CDI had higher observed mortality than other lineages, including ribotype 027, however.[85] Several studies have failed to observe any relationship between epidemic lineage CDI and severe clinical outcome.[86–88] Enhanced toxin production originally observed for epidemic lineage stains actually varies widely across strains of ribotype 027, and the significance of lineage with respect to clinical outcome has been cast into considerable question.[88–90] An association between epidemic lineage CDI and recurrence, however, has been consistently observed in many study settings.[91,92]

In 2005, severe CDI was reported in patients previously assumed to be at a low risk for CDI, including pregnant women and outpatients without known exposures to antimicrobials.[93] Population-based studies were subsequently undertaken that showed rates of community disease ranging between 6.9 and 23.4 cases per 100,000 person-years, but these were all based on laboratory surveillance.[94–97] These estimates of the incidence of community-acquired *C difficile* are far exceeded by incidence rates of hospital-acquired *C difficile*, which are approximately 5000 times higher. A subsequent study of the prevalence of CDI among community-dwellers testing positive for CDI in the evaluation of acute diarrheal syndromes showed that 43 of 1091 (3.9%) such patients tested positive for *C difficile*, but only three patients (0.3%) remained as possible CDI patients when more recognized causes of outpatient gastroenteritis, such as norovirus, were excluded.[98] CDI remains extremely unlikely as a cause of outpatient gastroenteritis based on available evidence.

Among patients with traditional risk factors for CDI (**Table 4**), several subgroups who experience exceptional rates of CDI have emerged, including solid organ transplant patients, bone marrow transplant patients, and patients with inflammatory bowel disease (Crohn's disease and ulcerative colitis) (**Table 5**). The rates of CDI observed in

Table 4
Clinical risk factors for CDI and recurrent CDI

Any Episode of CDI	Recurrent CDI
Age ≥65	Age 65
Length of inpatient stay	Number of prior CDI episodes
Antibiotic exposures • Clindamycin • Cephalosporins • Fluoroquinolones	Use of non-CDI antibiotics after CDI diagnosis
Proton pump inhibitors	Fluoroquinolone use Renal insufficiency Female gender NAP1/ribotype 027/BI/MLST1/*tcdC*1 lineage

these populations are readily expressed in denominators of 100, reflecting disease incidences 100 to 1000 times those observed in general inpatient populations and long-term care facilities. The unifying clinical feature of these groups is widespread use of broad-spectrum antimicrobials needed to manage conditions, such as febrile neutropenia and opportunistic infections, although all of these groups also share significant immunosuppression and exposure to health care facilities. Unfortunately, most clinical trials for CDI have traditionally excluded patients with underlying diarrheal disorders, such as inflammatory bowel disease, creating an evidence gap in the management of these patients. The impact of CDI on these populations is significant. In one study of kidney recipients, the attributable mortality of CDI was 0.7%, higher than the observed loss of transplant grafts because of thrombosis and rejection.[99] In a study of lung transplant recipients, 54% of CDI occurred within the first 6 months of transplant, and these early CDI patients had a higher risk of death.[100] In this cohort, 70% of CDI occurred after discharge from the initial hospitalization, such as in the outpatient setting or during readmissions for complications, rather than immediately postoperatively.[100]

The public health impact of CDI is substantial. The burden of CDI has been estimated at $2454 to $6326 in excess health care costs per case, resulting in additional US health care expenditures of $4.8 billion per year for acute care facilities alone.[101–103] Beyond the economic impact, *C difficile* results in an estimated 453,000

Table 5
Populations at exceptional risk for *Clostridium difficile* infection

Population	Prevalence (%)	Authors, References
Ulcerative colitis	3.7	Nguyen et al,[201] 2008
Crohn disease	1.1	Nguyen et al,[201] 2008
Kidney transplant	4.7	Paudel et al,[202] 2015
Pancreas transplant	3.2	Paudel et al,[202] 2015
Lung transplant	10.8	Paudel et al,[202] 2015
Liver transplant	9.1	Paudel et al,[202] 2015
Heart transplant	5.2	Paudel et al,[202] 2015
Solid organ transplant overall	7.4	Paudel et al,[202] 2015
Allogeneic bone marrow transplantation	8.4	Guddati et al,[203] 2014

cases and 29,000 deaths annually in the United States and has replaced methicillin-resistant *Staphylococcus aureus* as the most common cause of health care–associated infections in US hospitals.[104–106] In 2013, CDI was classified by the Centers for Disease Control and Prevention as one of three urgent antibiotic resistance threats in the United States that "require urgent public health attention to identify infections and to limit transmission."[107]

PATHOGENESIS

The secretory diarrhea and colonic inflammation seen in CDI is attributable to the effects of two large clostridial toxins, toxin A and toxin B, encoded by *tcdA* and *tcdB*, respectively, as part of the 19.6-kb pathogenicity locus (PaLoc) on the *C difficile* chromosome.[108–110] Nontoxigenic strains of *C difficile* in which the entire PaLoc is replaced with a 115-bp sequence are commonly encountered in colonized humans and the environment.[31,111] TcdA and TcdB, similar to other large clostridial toxins, glycosylate small guanosine triphosphatases in the Rho and Ras families when endocytosed into epithelial cells, leading to actin filament disassembly, disruption of tight junctions, and ultimately cell death.[112] Although toxin B is observed to intoxicate a wide variety of mammalian cell lines, candidate receptors responsible for cell surface binding and endocytosis in intestinal epithelial cells have only recently been characterized. Using an insertional mutagenesis technique in Caco-2 cells, LaFrance and colleagues[113] demonstrated that poliovirus receptor-like 3 is involved in binding of TcdB to its target, disruption of or pretreatment by antibodies to which creates resistance to toxin B in this cell line. Tao and colleagues,[114] however, failed to confirm this finding in HeLa or Caco-2 cells. Instead, their CRISPR-Cas9-mediated genome-wide screens identified members of the Wnt-binding frizzled family, particularly FZD1, 2, and 7, as the predominant receptors for TcdB. The finding that TcdB may compete directly with Wnt for FZD binding suggests that colonic epithelial disruption may be a direct consequence of TcdB, because Wnt signaling is particularly important for maintaining colonic stem cells.[114]

Previous studies using pure TcdB and TcdA pointed to a synergistic role for the two toxins in CDI, but the recent ability to create gene knockouts in *C difficile* has led to the demonstration that TcdB is necessary and sufficient to cause disease in the hamster and mouse models.[115,116] This finding is concordant with the clinical observation that TcdA−TcdB+ *C difficile* strains are fully capable of causing human disease.[117–119]

In wild-type strains of *C difficile*, *tcdA* and *tcdB* are expressed only in late-logarithmic and stationary growth phases.[109,120] Toxin production is under the immediate control of two other genes on the PaLoc, *tcdR* and *tcdC*, which serve as positive and negative regulators, respectively.[109,120–122] BI/NAP1/027 strains have been associated with nonsense mutations in *tcdC* that lead to a truncated, dysfunctional TcdC and thus TcdB production at all phases of growth, but these *tcdC* mutations are found in many other nonepidemic lineages.[25,123] There is also in vitro evidence that BI/NAP1/027 strains produce more toxins than wild-type strains, although many other lineages including the type stain VPI 10463 make substantially more toxin than epidemic lineages.[121,122,124]

C difficile also has potential virulence factors outside the PaLoc, including a binary toxin, encoded by two genes *cdtA* and *cdtB*, which is also prevalent among BI/NAP1/027 strains.[125–127] Evidence for a role of binary toxin in CDI, however, is limited by the observation that CDT+TcdA-TcdB- strains are incapable of reproducing CDI in the hamster model and that these strains have not yet been associated with human disease.[128] Preliminary evidence also points to increased adherence to intestinal mucosa mediated by mutations in *slpA*, a surface layer protein, in BI/NAP1/027 strains of *C difficile*.[129] BI/NAP1/027 strains may have an enhanced sporulation capacity compared with wild-type strains, but this finding has not been reproduced in later studies that have noted substantial variation within the epidemic lineage.[130,131] Antibiotic resistance, particularly to clindamycin, macrolides, fluoroquinolones, and rifampin, is also more common in the BI/NAP1/027 strains and leads to potentiation of the spread of the organism within hospitals where such antibiotics are in common use.[21,81,132]

The clear association of antibiotic use with CDI has focused attention on the relationship of the human microbiome to CDI risk. Using culture-independent 16S rRNA phylogenetic analysis of microbial components of stool flora, it was shown that the stool flora of patients with recurrent episodes of CDI were significantly less diverse than that of patients with initial episodes of CDI whose stool flora was, in turn, less diverse than control subjects.[133] In a subsequent study, pure culture of a single species of the Lachnospiraceae cultivated from mice that survived *C difficile* challenge were able to confer partial colonization resistance in a germ-free mouse model, although the mechanism for this colonization resistance was not determined.[134]

The role of conjugated primary bile salts (taurocholate and glycocholate) in recovering *C difficile* in the clinical microbiology laboratory has been known for some time[135]; early investigators hypothesized that the effect of antibiotics on the transit of these bile salts to the human large intestine after antibiotic use might be significant in the pathogenesis of CDI.[9,10] The significance of bile salts in the germination (by primary bile salts) and inhibition of *C difficile* outgrowth by chenodeoxycholate has recently been confirmed,[136,137] and subsequent studies in the mouse model of CDI correlated antibiotic challenge in mice with a shift from a predominance of deoxycholate, which inhibits *C difficile* outgrowth, to taurocholate, which is essential to germination, in the murine cecum.[138] Microbiome analysis of patients colonized with *C difficile* has suggested that *Clostridium scindens*, a bile acid 7α-dehydroxylating intestinal bacterium, is associated with resistance to CDI through its production of secondary bile acids,[139] a finding that awaits confirmation in formal trials of this candidate probiotic organism.

LABORATORY DIAGNOSIS

The laboratory diagnosis of CDI has undergone considerable upheaval since the first characterization of CDI. Cell culture cytotoxicity neutralization assays (CCCNAs) (see **Fig. 2**) were the only available clinical tests for CDI following the discovery of CDI; these tests recapitulate the process used to discover the disease. For CCCNAs, patient stool is filtered and incubated with human fibroblast cells with and without *C difficile* (originally *Clostridium sordellii*) antitoxin for up to 72 hours, and if the antitoxin-free well shows a cytopathic effect and the antitoxin well does not, the presence of *C difficile* toxin in stool is confirmed (see **Fig. 2**). CCCNA is technically demanding, takes 2 to 4 days to turn around a negative result, and is generally only performed by large clinical laboratories with the capacity to maintain cell cultures. Compared with identification of toxin-producing *C difficile* using anaerobic culture (termed toxigenic culture; discussed in the section on microbiology), CCCNA was observed to be 67% to 78% sensitive,[140,141] but the extent to which either CCCNA or toxigenic culture could be considered a reference standard was never established. Both CCCNA and toxigenic culture identify patients with colonization and are therefore susceptible to false positives for the end point of CDI. Eventually, CCCNA came to be regarded as a clinical gold standard in its own right to which more rapid immunoassays (EIA) were compared as they were introduced into clinical use in the 1980s.

Cell culture cytotoxicity assays were replaced by most clinical microbiology laboratories in North America and Europe by EIAs for TcdA or TcdA+TcdB because of their ease of use and rapid turnaround time of approximately 2 hours. Compared with CCCNA as a reference standard, EIA has a comparatively low sensitivity of 80% to 90%,[141–143] and it is even less sensitive when compared with toxigenic culture. Clinicians frequently sought to overcome the perceived sensitivity issue of immunoassays for CDI through use of repeated testing. Submission of multiple samples from the same patient within days became a common strategy for CCCNA and immunoassays, but these were observed to have a marginal return.[144–147] Various two-step testing algorithms incorporating a rapid antigen test for *C difficile* glutamate dehydrogenase (GDH) activity followed by reflex testing of positives to confirm toxin production by EIA or cell culture cytotoxicity were also devised,[148–150] but sensitivity of GDH screening varied by *C difficile* lineage, casting some doubt on this strategy.[151,152]

The introduction of nucleic acid testing for *C difficile* into clinical practice in 2008 (**Table 6**) initially held significant promise for improving the sensitivity of testing relative to EIA platforms and substantially reducing the turnaround time and technical complexity of CCCNA. The latest generation of molecular tests has emphasized the detection of *tcdB*, although platforms that are designed to detect only *tcdA* are still able to detect toxinA-/B+ strains because of a conserved fragment of *tcdA* present in these lineages. Almost all currently approved platforms incorporate sample lysis, DNA extraction, target amplification, and interpretation of internal controls into a single sample vessel or cartridge, substantially reducing the technical complexity of the tests compared with earlier generations of real-time PCR instruments. Assays based on toxin gene detection exclude false-positive results from detection of nontoxigenic strains of *C difficile*. The sensitivity of GDH antigen, PCR, and toxigenic culture were all recently shown to be decreased substantially by empiric therapy, with 45% of patients converting initially positive tests to negative within 3 days of therapy in one cohort of CDI patients.[153] The impact of empiric therapy has been poorly accounted for in most prior diagnostic test evaluations for CDI.

Recent studies of *C difficile* testing performance have focused on strategies to incorporate clinical outcome or symptoms into test performance given increasing concerns about the lack of specificity of laboratory diagnostics for CDI. Dubberke and colleagues[154] performed a prospective study of 150 patients being tested for CDI, including prospective evaluation of tested patients' symptoms using blinded physician

Table 6
Selected FDA-approved clinical diagnostic nucleic acid testing platforms for diagnosis of CDI

Device	Manufacturer	Approval	Platform	Gene Targets
Cobas	Roche	5/2015	RT-PCR	*tcdB*
BD MAX	BD Diagnostics	4/2013	RT-PCR	*tcdB*
Verigene	Nanosphere	12/2012	PCR + nanoparticle hybridization	*tcdA/tcdB/tcdC/cdt*
Simplexa	Focus	4/2012	RT-PCR	*tcdB*
Illumigene	Meridian	7/2010	LAMP	*tcdA*
Xpert	Cepheid	7/2009	RT-PCR	*tcdB/tcdC*
Progastro CD	Prodesse	4/2009	RT-PCR	*tcdB*
BD Geneohm	BD Diagnostics	12/2008	RT-PCR	*tcdB*

Abbreviations: FDA, Food and Drug Administration; RT-PCR, real-time PCR.

interviews as part of a reference standard for evaluating two different EIAs, three nucleic acid amplificiation tests, CCCNA, and toxigenic culture. Among the 150 patients, 44 were positive by toxigenic culture, but only 35 of these had clinically significant diarrhea.[154] Using a composite reference standard of four or more assays positive, 50 of 150 patients were positive, but only 40 of these patients had clinically significant diarrhea. As expected from prior studies, CCCNA had the lowest observed sensitivity regardless of reference standard used (55.0%–62.9%), whereas the nucleic acid tests had very high sensitivity (100%). Somewhat unexpectedly, the sensitivity of varying EIAs was actually higher than CCCNA, and the inclusion of clinical symptoms into the reference standard increased the specificity and positive predictive value of all tested assays. The authors observed that 15 patients whose diagnosis of CDI was rejected by EIA but positive by the composite reference standard (mostly by nucleic acid tests) had no diagnosis of CDI within 60 days despite 10 of 15 patients having clinically significant diarrhea and 4 of 15 patients receiving empiric therapy for CDI, suggesting that less sensitive tests like EIA may actually predict typical CDI features more reliably.[154] Planche and colleagues[155] conducted a much larger multicenter prospective observational study of 12,420 fecal samples from 6522 inpatient episodes of diarrhea. Mortality was observed in 72 of 435 (16.6%) patients with positive CCCNAs compared with 20 of 207 (9.7%) positive by toxigenic culture with negative CCCNAs and 503 of 5880 (8.6%) patients negative by both methods.[155] The authors also observed that patients with negative CCCNA but positive nucleic acid tests did not differ in their observed mortality, length of stay, or peak leukocyte count from patients negative on both assays; given that CDI is not 100% fatal this observation is not clearcut evidence that CCCNA remains the most relevant clinical standard for diagnosis, nor could algorithm combining EIA, GDH antigen, and nucleic acid testing fully replicate the sensitivity and specificity of CCCNA itself in their cohort.[155] Finally, Polage and colleagues[156] conducted a prospective cohort study at a single center of 1416 hospitalized adult patients tested for CDI using EIA and nucleic acid testing (PCR) during which the PCR results were withheld from ordering physicians. In this study 293 of 1416 (21%) were positive by PCR and 131 of 1416 (9.3%) were EIA-positive.[156] The authors observed that the EIA-/PCR+ patients had shorter duration of diarrhea than in EIA+/PCR+ patients despite minimal empiric treatment in the former group, and no CDI complications (attributable death, colectomy, intensive care unit stay) were observed versus 10 complications in patients with concordant tests.[156] Recurrent positive C difficile testing was observed in only 5 (3.1%) EIA-/PCR+ patients versus 14 (10.7%) of EIA+/PCR+ patients; deaths caused by recurrent CDI occurred in both groups, but at significantly lower rates in the EIA-/PCR+ group.[156] The study did not include prospective use of CCCNA or toxigenic culture as a reference standard, however, which may have misclassified patients in the EIA-/PCR- group with mild CDI as control group patients, but overall this study adds to a body of evidence that nucleic acid tests may substantially overdiagnose CDI. The available evidence, however, does not yet support that a return to EIA as the principal diagnostic test for CDI would not result in significant loss of sensitivity for diagnosis of patients with mild CDI. The need for laboratory correlates of colonization versus infection remains acute, and CDI will remain partly a clinical diagnosis until additional diagnostics are developed (discussed in the section on differential diagnosis).

TREATMENT, PROGNOSIS, AND LONG-TERM OUTCOME

Before recent shifts in observed incidence and severity after 2001, CDI was often regarded as a self-limited disease so long as the inciting antimicrobial agents could be stopped. Early therapeutic trials sometimes contained placebo arms, and head-to-head comparisons of the two main *C difficile* antimicrobials, enteral vancomycin and metronidazole, failed to show superiority for either.[157] Metronidazole was generally recommended by expert guidelines as first-line therapy for reasons of cost and out of concern that widespread use of vancomycin would promote acquisition of vancomycin-resistant enterococci.[158] A randomized, double-blind trial of metronidazole versus vancomycin, however, showed superior response rates for vancomycin in a subset of patients with severe disease.[159] Metronidazole was also found to be inferior to vancomycin for the end point of clinical success (defined as cessation of diarrhea for ≥ 2 days) in all patients with CDI in a multisite blinded, randomized trial with 72.7% versus 81.1% success rates observed, respectively.[160] Fidaxomicin, a new macrocyclic antimicrobial, was observed to be noninferior to vancomycin in three randomized trials, but it did not demonstrate superiority for the end point of clinical success. Although much has been made of the observation that fidaxomicin has an approximately 10% reduced risk for recurrence compared with vancomycin, this was not consistent across studies and not tested in patients with multiple CDI recurrences, who were excluded from these trials.[161–163] Current clinical guidelines stress the use of vancomycin monotherapy for patients observed to be at risk for severe disease based on varying clinical criteria, although metronidazole use in patients with milder CDI is still recommended.[164,165]

The debates regarding which anti–*C difficile* antimicrobial is preferred in CDI management have been largely eclipsed by the observation of high rates of success for management of CDI, particularly multiply recurrent cases, with fecal microbiota transplantation (FMT).[166–171] In contrast to defined probiotic formulations, high-quality evidence has emerged showing that FMT is superior to vancomycin in management of recurrent CDI (**Table 7**). The regulatory status of FMT with the Food and Drug Administration remains uncertain, however, and the risk of short- and long-term donor-derived infection, particularly in immunosuppressed patients with CDI, remains a concern for this treatment modality. The optimal dose, route of delivery, and donor source for FMT have yet to be determined in well-controlled randomized trials, as is the use of FMT for first episodes of CDI. The risks of nondisclosure of sexual risk-taking and self-reported diarrheal illness in paid FMT donors and the use of small numbers of FMT donors for large numbers of recipients for the sake of improved patient access to this treatment modality may prove to be short-sighted in assessing the long-term risks of FMT in transmission of undiscovered pathogens. Nonetheless, FMT has emerged as the most effective single therapy for management of patients with recurrent CDI.

The prognosis for most patients with CDI remains favorable, but adverse event rates for CDI (colectomy/death) reached 44 of 253 (17.3%) for inpatients with hospital-acquired CDI at the University of Pittsburgh during a 2-year period.[82] A 30-day attributable mortality of 6.9% was observed in 20 hospitals in Quebec subsequently.[81] For patients who require colectomy, all-cause mortality is 50%.[67] Recently, surgical interventions have been devised that allow for delivery of vancomycin to the cecum of patients with severe, fulminant CDI using a loop ileostomy technique; this has substantially improved observed success rates compared with historical control subjects who underwent colectomy.[172]

DIFFERENTIAL DIAGNOSIS

The high prevalence of *C difficile* colonization among inpatients and more modest colonization among outpatients often obscures several infectious and noninfectious

Table 7
Key trials of FMT for treatment of recurrent CDI

N =	Design	Comparator	Dose (Estimated Stool Mass)	Route	Follow-up	Observed Successes (Per Protocol)	Comments	Authors, References
42	Randomized open label	Vancomycin ± laxative	500 mL (~50 g)	Nasoduodenal tube	10 wk	13/16 (81%) single dose 15/16 (94%) overall 7/26 (27%) patients in comparator arms	3 patients required second dose	van Nood et al,[169] 2013
20	Open label	None	48 g	Oral capsules (n = 30)	8 wk	14/20 single dosing 19/20 second dose	15 capsules × 2 d = 1 dose	Youngster et al,[170] 2014
20	Randomized nastogastric tube vs colonoscopy	None	90 mL (41 g)	Nasogastric tube Colonoscopy	8 wk	8/10 colonoscopic 6/10 nasogastric tube	All unrelated donors Nonsignificant difference in success	Youngster et al,[171] 2014
80	Retrospective multicenter case series	None	Varied	Colonoscopy	12 wk	62/80 (78%) single dose 70/80 (89%) multiple doses	First series to report inclusion of immunocompromised (n = 19 organ transplants, 3 HIV+)	Kelly et al,[167] 2014
43	Case series, directed fresh donors vs standardized frozen donors	None	250 mL (50 g)	Colonoscopy	8 wk	7/10 directed 30/33 stoolbank $P = .12$	30% inflammatory bowel disease Unrelated donors from stool bank	Hamilton et al,[166] 2012
46	Randomized controlled double-blind	Autologous stool (recipient's)	300 mL (64 g)	Colonoscopy	8 wk	22/22 (90.9%) donor FMT 15/24 (62.5%) autologous FMT	IBD and age ≥75 patients excluded 90% success for autologous stool reported at a single center	Kelly et al,[168] 2016
219	Randomized, double-blind frozen vs fresh FMT dose	None	50 mL (12.5 g)	Retention enema	13 wk	76/91 (83.5%) frozen FMT 74/87 (85.1%) fresh FMT	Single dose response rates much lower (62%–63%)	Lee et al,[204] 2016

Abbreviations: HIV, human immunodeficiency virus; IBD, inflammatory bowel disease.

causes of diarrhea and gastroenteritis when a positive *C difficile* diagnostic test is generated, resulting in substantial diagnostic test bias. Among outpatients presenting with acute gastroenteritis, particularly with vomiting, norovirus remains the most prevalent cause. Most new molecular diagnostic platforms that are replacing stool cultures for routine enteric pathogens in clinical microbiology laboratories are incorporating tests for not only *C difficile* but also norovirus, astrovirus, sapovirus, and others. Most patients without traditional risk factors for CDI who test positive for a viral cause and *C difficile* are probably colonized with the latter, and treatment of *C difficile* in these patients should be avoided. Treatment with vancomycin has been observed to prolong carriage with toxigenic *C difficile* and, in one instance, to actually provoke CDI in a patient with previously asymptomatic carriage.[173]

Among inpatients who present with diarrhea greater than 3 calendar days after admission, CDI is widely cited as the most prevalent infectious cause. With the increasing focus on early and aggressive diagnosis of CDI, however, it is often overlooked that noninfectious causes of diarrhea predominate, particularly postantibiotic diarrhea not associated with *C difficile*. Osmotic diarrhea from enteral feeding formulations, malabsorption related to ischemic colitis, and inflammatory diarrhea from ulcerative colitis and Crohn disease should always be considered in the differential diagnosis for diarrheal illnesses presenting in hospitalized patients. Even laxative use has been observed in 20% of hospitalized patients being tested for CDI, however,[154] and the rate of diagnoses other than CDI was greater than 90% in the largest diagnostic testing cohort yet reported,[155] indicating that CDI remains an uncommon finding among hospitalized patients with diarrhea. Patients with any of these causes of diarrhea are frequently colonized with *C difficile* and are found on diagnostic testing, and to date there is no laboratory assay that can distinguish colonization from CDI. Fecal leukocytes, fecal calprotectin levels, and C-reactive protein have all been proposed as biomarkers to make this distinction, but none of these can distinguish CDI from inflammatory bowel disease flares.[174,175] Thus, the diagnosis of CDI remains partly a clinical one. The absence of known risk factors, intact serum albumin levels, normal peripheral leukocyte counts, and a failure to exhibit any improvement after 10 days of antimicrobial therapy for CDI should raise suspicion that a patient with a positive *C difficile* stool test does not have CDI.

In the era of FMT, making the distinction between colonization and CDI is particularly important; patients with alternate causes of diarrhea are highly unlikely to benefit from FMT based on available data. In one outpatient study of 117 patients referred 2013 to 2014 to an FMT clinic, 29 patients (25%) were determined to have an alternative diagnosis, most frequently irritable bowel syndrome.[176] Because many patients with a history of multiple positive *C difficile* tests may have had inappropriate tests of cure while experiencing irritable bowel syndrome after recovery from CDI, careful history-taking must distinguish patients who exhibit a pattern of worsening symptoms days to weeks after cessation of CDI antibiotics from those who have "refractory CDI" regardless of their treatment status. Although common in clinical parlance, "chronic," "treatment-refractory," and "treatment-resistant" CDI is unlikely to exist based on available evidence, and the preponderance of the of patients in CDI clinical trials who "fail" vancomycin and fidaxomicin (~ 10% in most recent trials) are probably among the patients who did not have CDI given the low observed mortality among these patients.

IMMUNITY AND REINFECTION

The most troubling aspect of CDI is the high relapse rate of 10% to 35% after a first episode, approximately 40% after a first recurrence, and 60% to 100% following two or more recurrences.[177] Patients with multiple CDI have been strongly associated with a failure to demonstrate an anamnestic IgG response against TcdA.[178–182] Besides age and immune senescence, continued exposure to antibiotics is a powerful predictor of CDI relapse.[183] Efforts to devise a *C difficile* toxoid vaccine have met with initial success in individuals with multiple relapses,[184] but to date there are no published trials using vaccines for primary prevention of CDI. The debilitating effects of multiple CDI relapses were the principal drivers of the development of FMT, which has emerged as the only reliable treatment modality to date. A randomized, placebo-controlled trial of passive immunotherapy for recurrent CDI using monoclonal antibodies to TcdA and TcdB showed an 18% reduction in the absolute risk of recurrence.[185] Two phase 3 evaluations of these antibodies revealed that the antibody to TcdB (bezlotoxumab) was the active component, reducing recurrence rates by 10% compared with placebo.[186,187] Bezlotoxumab is available only parenterally, must be used with standard antimicrobial therapies for CDI, and is likely to be substantially more costly than (and likely less effective than) FMT in managing recurrent CDI, however, and its role in clinical care of patients with CDI has yet to be established.

SUMMARY

CDIs have emerged as one of the principal threats to the health of hospitalized and immunocompromised patients. Nucleic acid testing for *C difficile* toxin genes has eclipsed traditional clinical diagnostics for CDI in sensitivity and is now widespread in clinical use, but preliminary evidence suggests that this may have come at a cost of substantially reduced positive predictive value. The importance of *C difficile* colonization is increasingly recognized not only as a source for false-positive clinical testing but also as a source of new infections within hospitals and other health care environments. In the last 5 years, FMT has emerged as the most effective treatment of patients with multiply recurrent CDI. The increasing understanding of the microbiome and colonization resistance as one of the host defenses against CDI will likely result in improved therapeutics for CDI in the next decade.

REFERENCES

1. Hall I, O'Toole E. Intestinal flora in newborn infants with a description of a new pathogenic anaerobe, *Bacillus difficilis*. Am J Dis Child 1935;49:390–402.
2. Bartlett JG, Chang TW, Gurwith M, et al. Antibiotic-associated pseudomembranous colitis due to toxin-producing clostridia. N Engl J Med 1978;298(10):531–4.
3. Bartlett JG, Onderdonk AB, Cisneros RL, et al. Clindamycin-associated colitis due to a toxin-producing species of *Clostridium* in hamsters. J Infect Dis 1977;136(5):701–5.
4. Jump RL, Pultz MJ, Donskey CJ. Vegetative *Clostridium difficile* survives in room air on moist surfaces and in gastric contents with reduced acidity: a potential mechanism to explain the association between proton pump inhibitors and *C difficile*-associated diarrhea? Antimicrob Agents Chemother 2007;51(8):2883–7.
5. Arroyo LG, Rousseau J, Willey BM, et al. Use of a selective enrichment broth to recover *Clostridium difficile* from stool swabs stored under different conditions. J Clin Microbiol 2005;43(10):5341–3.
6. Riggs MM, Sethi AK, Zabarsky TF, et al. Asymptomatic carriers are a potential source for transmission of epidemic and nonepidemic *Clostridium difficile* strains among long-term care facility residents. Clin Infect Dis 2007;45(8):992–8.

7. Hink T, Burnham CA, Dubberke ER. A systematic evaluation of methods to optimize culture-based recovery of *Clostridium difficile* from stool specimens. Anaerobe 2013;19:39–43.

8. Jackson S, Calos M, Myers A, et al. Analysis of proline reduction in the nosocomial pathogen *Clostridium difficile*. J Bacteriol 2006;188(24):8487–95.

9. Wilson KH. Efficiency of various bile salt preparations for stimulation of *Clostridium difficile* spore germination. J Clin Microbiol 1983;18(4):1017–9.

10. Wilson KH, Kennedy MJ, Fekety FR. Use of sodium taurocholate to enhance spore recovery on a medium selective for *Clostridium difficile*. J Clin Microbiol 1982;15(3):443–6.

11. Dawson LF, Stabler RA, Wren BW. Assessing the role of p-cresol tolerance in *Clostridium difficile*. J Med Microbiol 2008;57(Pt 6):745–9.

12. Sivsammye G, Sims HV. Presumptive identification of *Clostridium difficile* by detection of p-cresol in prepared peptone yeast glucose broth supplemented with p-hydroxyphenylacetic acid. J Clin Microbiol 1990;28(8):1851–3.

13. Fedorko DP, Williams EC. Use of cycloserine-cefoxitin-fructose agar and L-proline-aminopeptidase (PRO Discs) in the rapid identification of *Clostridium difficile*. J Clin Microbiol 1997;35(5):1258–9.

14. Chen JH, Cheng VC, Wong OY, et al. The importance of matrix-assisted laser desorption ionization-time of flight mass spectrometry for correct identification of *Clostridium difficile* isolated from chromID *C difficile* chromogenic agar. J Microbiol Immunol Infect 2016. [Epub ahead of print].

15. Coltella L, Mancinelli L, Onori M, et al. Advancement in the routine identification of anaerobic bacteria by MALDI-TOF mass spectrometry. Eur J Clin Microbiol Infect Dis 2013;32(9):1183–92.

16. Kim YJ, Kim SH, Park HJ, et al. MALDI-TOF MS is more accurate than VITEK II ANC card and API Rapid ID 32 A system for the identification of *Clostridium* species. Anaerobe 2016;40:73–5.

17. Edwards AN, McBride SM. Isolating and purifying *Clostridium difficile* spores. Methods Mol Biol 2016;1476:117–28.

18. Perez J, Springthorpe VS, Sattar SA. Clospore: a liquid medium for producing high titers of semi-purified spores of *Clostridium difficile*. J AOAC Int 2011; 94(2):618–26.

19. Bouillaut L, Dubois T, Sonenshein AL, et al. Integration of metabolism and virulence in *Clostridium difficile*. Res Microbiol 2015;166(4):375–83.

20. Darkoh C, Dupont HL, Kaplan HB. Novel one-step method for detection and isolation of active-toxin-producing *Clostridium difficile* strains directly from stool samples. J Clin Microbiol 2011;49(12):4219–24.

21. McDonald LC, Killgore GE, Thompson A, et al. An epidemic, toxin gene-variant strain of *Clostridium difficile*. N Engl J Med 2005;353(23):2433–41.

22. Corkill JE, Graham R, Hart CA, et al. Pulsed-field gel electrophoresis of degradation-sensitive DNAs from *Clostridium difficile* PCR ribotype 1 strains. J Clin Microbiol 2000;38(7):2791–2.

23. Stubbs SL, Brazier JS, O'Neill GL, et al. PCR targeted to the 16S-23S rRNA gene intergenic spacer region of *Clostridium difficile* and construction of a library consisting of 116 different PCR ribotypes. J Clin Microbiol 1999;37(2):461–3.

24. Griffiths D, Fawley W, Kachrimanidou M, et al. Multilocus sequence typing of *Clostridium difficile*. J Clin Microbiol 2010;48(3):770–8.

25. Curry SR, Marsh JW, Muto CA, et al. *tcdC* genotypes associated with severe TcdC truncation in an epidemic clone and other strains of *Clostridium difficile*. J Clin Microbiol 2007;45(1):215–21.

26. Dingle KE, Griffiths D, Didelot X, et al. Clinical *Clostridium difficile*: clonality and pathogenicity locus diversity. PLoS One 2011;6(5):e19993.

27. Clabots CR, Johnson S, Bettin KM, et al. Development of a rapid and efficient restriction endonuclease analysis typing system for *Clostridium difficile* and correlation with other typing systems. J Clin Microbiol 1993;31(7):1870–5.

28. Eyre DW, Cule ML, Wilson DJ, et al. Diverse sources of *C difficile* infection identified on whole-genome sequencing. N Engl J Med 2013;369(13):1195–205.

29. Marsh JW, O'Leary MM, Shutt KA, et al. Multilocus variable-number tandem-repeat analysis for investigation of *Clostridium difficile* transmission in Hospitals. J Clin Microbiol 2006;44(7):2558–66.

30. van den Berg RJ, Schaap I, Templeton KE, et al. Typing and subtyping of *Clostridium difficile* isolates by using multiple-locus variable-number tandem-repeat analysis. J Clin Microbiol 2007;45(3):1024–8.

31. al Saif N, Brazier JS. The distribution of *Clostridium difficile* in the environment of South Wales. J Med Microbiol 1996;45(2):133–7.

32. Moono P, Foster NF, Hampson DJ, et al. *Clostridium difficile* infection in production animals and avian species: a review. Foodborne Pathog Dis 2016;13(12): 647–55.

33. Hammitt MC, Bueschel DM, Keel MK, et al. A possible role for *Clostridium difficile* in the etiology of calf enteritis. Vet Microbiol 2008;127(3–4):343–52.

34. Larson HE, Price AB, Honour P, et al. *Clostridium difficile* and the aetiology of pseudomembranous colitis. Lancet 1978;1(8073):1063–6.

35. Sun X, Wang H, Zhang Y, et al. Mouse relapse model of *Clostridium difficile* infection. Infect Immun 2011;79(7):2856–64.

36. Curry SR, Marsh JW, Schlackman JL, et al. Prevalence of *Clostridium difficile* in uncooked ground meat products from Pittsburgh, Pennsylvania. Appl Environ Microbiol 2012;78(12):4183–6.

37. Weese JS, Avery BP, Rousseau J, et al. Detection and enumeration of *Clostridium difficile* spores in retail beef and pork. Appl Environ Microbiol 2009; 75(15):5009–11.

38. Marsh JW. Counterpoint: is *Clostridium difficile* a food-borne disease? Anaerobe 2013;21:62–3.

39. Marsh JW, Tulenko MM, Shutt KA, et al. Multi-locus variable number tandem repeat analysis for investigation of the genetic association of *Clostridium difficile* isolates from food, food animals and humans. Anaerobe 2011;17(4):156–60.

40. Jury LA, Sitzlar B, Kundrapu S, et al. Outpatient healthcare settings and transmission of *Clostridium difficile*. PLoS One 2013;8(7):e70175.

41. Kim KH, Fekety R, Batts DH, et al. Isolation of *Clostridium difficile* from the environment and contacts of patients with antibiotic-associated colitis. J Infect Dis 1981;143(1):42–50.

42. Fawley WN, Underwood S, Freeman J, et al. Efficacy of hospital cleaning agents and germicides against epidemic *Clostridium difficile* strains. Infect Control Hosp Epidemiol 2007;28(8):920–5.

43. Lawley TD, Clare S, Deakin LJ, et al. Use of purified *Clostridium difficile* spores to facilitate evaluation of health care disinfection regimens. Appl Environ Microbiol 2010;76(20):6895–900.

44. Perez J, Springthorpe VS, Sattar SA. Activity of selected oxidizing microbicides against the spores of *Clostridium difficile*: relevance to environmental control. Am J Infect Control 2005;33(6):320–5.

45. Shaughnessy MK, Micielli RL, DePestel DD, et al. Evaluation of hospital room assignment and acquisition of *Clostridium difficile* infection. Infect Control Hosp Epidemiol 2011;32(3):201–6.

46. Freedberg DE, Salmasian H, Cohen B, et al. Receipt of antibiotics in hospitalized patients and risk for *Clostridium difficile* infection in subsequent patients who occupy the same bed. JAMA Intern Med 2016;176(12):1801–8.

47. Muto CA, Blank MK, Marsh JW, et al. Control of an outbreak of infection with the hypervirulent *Clostridium difficile* BI strain in a university hospital using a comprehensive "bundle" approach. Clin Infect Dis 2007;45(10):1266–73.

48. Deshpande A, Mana TS, Cadnum JL, et al. Evaluation of a sporicidal peracetic acid/hydrogen peroxide-based daily disinfectant cleaner. Infect Control Hosp Epidemiol 2014;35(11):1414–6.

49. Nerandzic MM, Cadnum JL, Pultz MJ, et al. Evaluation of an automated ultraviolet radiation device for decontamination of *Clostridium difficile* and other healthcare-associated pathogens in hospital rooms. BMC Infect Dis 2010;10: 197.

50. Davies A, Pottage T, Bennett A, et al. Gaseous and air decontamination technologies for *Clostridium difficile* in the healthcare environment. J Hosp Infect 2011; 77(3):199–203.

51. Levin J, Riley LS, Parrish C, et al. The effect of portable pulsed xenon ultraviolet light after terminal cleaning on hospital-associated *Clostridium difficile* infection in a community hospital. Am J Infect Control 2013;41(8):746–8.

52. Miller R, Simmons S, Dale C, et al. Utilization and impact of a pulsed-xenon ultraviolet room disinfection system and multidisciplinary care team on *Clostridium difficile* in a long-term acute care facility. Am J Infect Control 2015; 43(12):1350–3.

53. Boyce JM, Havill NL, Otter JA, et al. Impact of hydrogen peroxide vapor room decontamination on *Clostridium difficile* environmental contamination and transmission in a healthcare setting. Infect Control Hosp Epidemiol 2008;29(8): 723–9.

54. Bouza E, Martin A, Van den Berg RJ, et al. Laboratory-acquired *Clostridium difficile* polymerase chain reaction ribotype 027: a new risk for laboratory workers? Clin Infect Dis 2008;47(11):1493–4.

55. Nakamura S, Mikawa M, Nakashio S, et al. Isolation of *Clostridium difficile* from the feces and the antibody in sera of young and elderly adults. Microbiol Immunol 1981;25(4):345–51.

56. Ozaki E, Kato H, Kita H, et al. *Clostridium difficile* colonization in healthy adults: transient colonization and correlation with enterococcal colonization. J Med Microbiol 2004;53(Pt 2):167–72.

57. Galdys AL, Nelson JS, Shutt KA, et al. Prevalence and duration of asymptomatic *Clostridium difficile* carriage among healthy subjects in Pittsburgh, Pennsylvania. J Clin Microbiol 2014;52(7):2406–9.

58. McFarland LV, Mulligan ME, Kwok RY, et al. Nosocomial acquisition of *Clostridium difficile* infection. N Engl J Med 1989;320(4):204–10.

59. Clabots CR, Johnson S, Olson MM, et al. Acquisition of *Clostridium difficile* by hospitalized patients: evidence for colonized new admissions as a source of infection. J Infect Dis 1992;166(3):561–7.

60. Lanzas C, Dubberke ER, Lu Z, et al. Epidemiological model for *Clostridium difficile* transmission in healthcare settings. Infect Control Hosp Epidemiol 2011; 32(6):553–61.

61. Curry SR, Muto CA, Schlackman JL, et al. Use of multilocus variable number of tandem repeats analysis genotyping to determine the role of asymptomatic carriers in *Clostridium difficile* transmission. Clin Infect Dis 2013;57(8):1094–102.

62. Loo VG, Bourgault AM, Poirier L, et al. Host and pathogen factors for *Clostridium difficile* infection and colonization. N Engl J Med 2011;365(18):1693–703.

63. Longtin Y, Paquet-Bolduc B, Gilca R, et al. Effect of detecting and isolating *Clostridium difficile* carriers at hospital admission on the incidence of *C difficile* infections: a Quasi-experimental controlled study. JAMA Intern Med 2016;176(6): 796–804.

64. Manabe YC, Vinetz JM, Moore RD, et al. *Clostridium difficile* colitis: an efficient clinical approach to diagnosis. Ann Intern Med 1995;123(11):835–40.

65. Wanahita A, Goldsmith EA, Marino BJ, et al. *Clostridium difficile* infection in patients with unexplained leukocytosis. Am J Med 2003;115(7):543–6.

66. Wanahita A, Goldsmith EA, Musher DM. Conditions associated with leukocytosis in a tertiary care hospital, with particular attention to the role of infection caused by *Clostridium difficile*. Clin Infect Dis 2002;34(12):1585–92.

67. Dallal RM, Harbrecht BG, Boujoukas AJ, et al. Fulminant *Clostridium difficile*: an underappreciated and increasing cause of death and complications. Ann Surg 2002;235(3):363–72.

68. Fujitani S, George WL, Murthy AR. Comparison of clinical severity score indices for *Clostridium difficile* infection. Infect Control Hosp Epidemiol 2011;32(3): 220–8.

69. Na X, Martin AJ, Sethi S, et al. A multi-center prospective derivation and validation of a clinical prediction tool for severe *Clostridium difficile* infection. PLoS One 2015;10(4):e0123405.

70. Miller MA, Louie T, Mullane K, et al. Derivation and validation of a simple clinical bedside score (ATLAS) for *Clostridium difficile* infection which predicts response to therapy. BMC Infect Dis 2013;13:148.

71. Hu MY, Katchar K, Kyne L, et al. Prospective derivation and validation of a clinical prediction rule for recurrent *Clostridium difficile* infection. Gastroenterology 2009;136(4):1206–14.

72. Villano SA, Seiberling M, Tatarowicz W, et al. Evaluation of an oral suspension of VP20621, spores of nontoxigenic *Clostridium difficile* strain M3, in healthy subjects. Antimicrob Agents Chemother 2012;56(10):5224–9.

73. Samore MH, DeGirolami PC, Tlucko A, et al. *Clostridium difficile* colonization and diarrhea at a tertiary care hospital. Clin Infect Dis 1994;18(2):181–7.

74. Shim JK, Johnson S, Samore MH, et al. Primary symptomless colonisation by *Clostridium difficile* and decreased risk of subsequent diarrhoea. Lancet 1998;351(9103):633–6.

75. Kutty PK, Benoit SR, Woods CW, et al. Assessment of *Clostridium difficile*-associated disease surveillance definitions, North Carolina, 2005. Infect Control Hosp Epidemiol 2008;29(3):197–202.

76. McDonald LC, Coignard B, Dubberke E, et al. Recommendations for surveillance of *Clostridium difficile*-associated disease. Infect Control Hosp Epidemiol 2007;28(2):140–5.

77. Kelly CP, Pothoulakis C, LaMont JT. *Clostridium difficile* colitis. N Engl J Med 1994;330(4):257–62.

78. Brown E, Talbot GH, Axelrod P, et al. Risk factors for *Clostridium difficile* toxin-associated diarrhea. Infect Control Hosp Epidemiol 1990;11(6):283–90.

79. McDonald LC, Owings M, Jernigan DB. *Clostridium difficile* infection in patients discharged from US short-stay hospitals, 1996-2003. Emerg Infect Dis 2006; 12(3):409–15.

80. Zilberberg MD, Shorr AF, Kollef MH. Increase in adult *Clostridium difficile*-related hospitalizations and case-fatality rate, United States, 2000-2005. Emerg Infect Dis 2008;14(6):929–31.

81. Loo VG, Poirier L, Miller MA, et al. A predominantly clonal multi-institutional outbreak of *Clostridium difficile*-associated diarrhea with high morbidity and mortality. N Engl J Med 2005;353(23):2442–9.

82. Muto CA, Pokrywka M, Shutt K, et al. A large outbreak of *Clostridium difficile*-associated disease with an unexpected proportion of deaths and colectomies at a teaching hospital following increased fluoroquinolone use. Infect Control Hosp Epidemiol 2005;26(3):273–80.

83. Rupnik M, Wilcox MH, Gerding DN. *Clostridium difficile* infection: new developments in epidemiology and pathogenesis. Nat Rev Microbiol 2009;7(7):526–36.

84. See I, Mu Y, Cohen J, et al. NAP1 strain type predicts outcomes from *Clostridium difficile* infection. Clin Infect Dis 2014;58(10):1394–400.

85. Walker AS, Eyre DW, Wyllie DH, et al. Relationship between bacterial strain type, host biomarkers, and mortality in *Clostridium difficile* infection. Clin Infect Dis 2013;56(11):1589–600.

86. Sirard S, Valiquette L, Fortier LC. Lack of association between clinical outcome of *Clostridium difficile* infections, strain type, and virulence-associated phenotypes. J Clin Microbiol 2011;49(12):4040–6.

87. Cloud J, Noddin L, Pressman A, et al. *Clostridium difficile* strain NAP-1 is not associated with severe disease in a nonepidemic setting. Clin Gastroenterol Hepatol 2009;7(8):868–73.e2.

88. Walk ST, Micic D, Jain R, et al. *Clostridium difficile* ribotype does not predict severe infection. Clin Infect Dis 2012;55(12):1661–8.

89. Carlson PE Jr, Walk ST, Bourgis AE, et al. The relationship between phenotype, ribotype, and clinical disease in human *Clostridium difficile* isolates. Anaerobe 2013;24:109–16.

90. Aitken SL, Alam MJ, Khaleduzzaman M, et al. In the endemic setting, *Clostridium difficile* ribotype 027 is virulent but not hypervirulent. Infect Control Hosp Epidemiol 2015;36(11):1318–23.

91. Marsh JW, Arora R, Schlackman JL, et al. Association of relapse of *Clostridium difficile* disease with BI/NAP1/027. J Clin Microbiol 2012;50(12):4078–82.

92. Petrella LA, Sambol SP, Cheknis A, et al. Decreased cure and increased recurrence rates for *Clostridium difficile* infection caused by the epidemic *C difficile* BI strain. Clin Infect Dis 2012;55(3):351–7.

93. Centers for Disease Control and Prevention (CDC). Severe *Clostridium difficile*-associated disease in populations previously at low risk–four states, 2005. MMWR Morb Mortal Wkly Rep 2005;54(47):1201–5.

94. Centers for Disease Control and Prevention (CDC). Surveillance for community-associated *Clostridium difficile*-Connecticut, 2006. MMWR Morb Mortal Wkly Rep 2008;57(13):340–3.

95. Lambert PJ, Dyck M, Thompson LH, et al. Population-based surveillance of *Clostridium difficile* infection in Manitoba, Canada, by using interim surveillance definitions. Infect Control Hosp Epidemiol 2009;30(10):945–51.

96. Kutty PK, Woods CW, Sena AC, et al. Risk factors for and estimated incidence of community-associated *Clostridium difficile* infection, North Carolina, USA. Emerg Infect Dis 2010;16(2):197–204.

97. Fellmeth G, Yarlagadda S, Iyer S. Epidemiology of community-onset *Clostridium difficile* infection in a community in the South of England. J Infect Public Health 2010;3(3):118–23.

98. Hirshon JM, Thompson AD, Limbago B, et al. *Clostridium difficile* infection in outpatients, Maryland and Connecticut, USA, 2002-2007. Emerg Infect Dis 2011;17(10):1946–9.

99. Mitu-Pretorian OM, Forgacs B, Qumruddin A, et al. Outcomes of patients who develop symptomatic *Clostridium difficile* infection after solid organ transplantation. Transplant Proc 2010;42(7):2631–3.

100. Lee JT, Kelly RF, Hertz MI, et al. *Clostridium difficile* infection increases mortality risk in lung transplant recipients. J Heart Lung Transplant 2013;32(10):1020–6.

101. Dubberke ER, Olsen MA. Burden of *Clostridium difficile* on the healthcare system. Clin Infect Dis 2012;55(Suppl 2):S88–92.

102. Dubberke ER, Reske KA, Olsen MA, et al. Short- and long-term attributable costs of *Clostridium difficile*-associated disease in nonsurgical inpatients. Clin Infect Dis 2008;46(4):497–504.

103. Kyne L, Hamel MB, Polavaram R, et al. Health care costs and mortality associated with nosocomial diarrhea due to *Clostridium difficile*. Clin Infect Dis 2002; 34(3):346–53.

104. Lessa FC, Winston LG, McDonald LC, et al. Burden of *Clostridium difficile* infection in the United States. N Engl J Med 2015;372(24):2369–70.

105. Magill SS, Edwards JR, Bamberg W, et al. Multistate point-prevalence survey of health care-associated infections. N Engl J Med 2014;370(13):1198–208.

106. Miller BA, Chen LF, Sexton DJ, et al. Comparison of the burdens of hospital-onset, healthcare facility-associated *Clostridium difficile* Infection and of healthcare-associated infection due to methicillin-resistant *Staphylococcus aureus* in community hospitals. Infect Control Hosp Epidemiol 2011;32(4): 387–90.

107. CDC. Antibiotic resistance threats in the United States. 2013. Available at: http://www.cdc.gov/drugresistance/threat-report-2013/pdf/ar-threats-2013-508.pdf. Accessed November 11, 2016.

108. Braun V, Hundsberger T, Leukel P, et al. Definition of the single integration site of the pathogenicity locus in *Clostridium difficile*. Gene 1996;181(1–2):29–38.

109. Hundsberger T, Braun V, Weidmann M, et al. Transcription analysis of the genes tcdA-E of the pathogenicity locus of *Clostridium difficile*. Eur J Biochem 1997; 244(3):735–42.

110. Soehn F, Wagenknecht-Wiesner A, Leukel P, et al. Genetic rearrangements in the pathogenicity locus of *Clostridium difficile* strain 8864: implications for transcription, expression and enzymatic activity of toxins A and B. Mol Gen Genet 1998;258(3):222–32.

111. Cohen SH, Tang YJ, Silva J Jr. Analysis of the pathogenicity locus in *Clostridium difficile* strains. J Infect Dis 2000;181(2):659–63.

112. Voth DE, Ballard JD. *Clostridium difficile* toxins: mechanism of action and role in disease. Clin Microbiol Rev 2005;18(2):247–63.

113. LaFrance ME, Farrow MA, Chandrasekaran R, et al. Identification of an epithelial cell receptor responsible for *Clostridium difficile* TcdB-induced cytotoxicity. Proc Natl Acad Sci U S A 2015;112(22):7073–8.

114. Tao L, Zhang J, Meraner P, et al. Frizzled proteins are colonic epithelial receptors for *C difficile* toxin B. Nature 2016;538(7625):350–5.

115. Lyras D, O'Connor JR, Howarth PM, et al. Toxin B is essential for virulence of *Clostridium difficile*. Nature 2009;458(7242):1176–9.

116. Carter GP, Chakravorty A, Pham Nguyen TA, et al. Defining the roles of TcdA and TcdB in localized gastrointestinal disease, systemic organ damage, and the host response during *Clostridium difficile* infections. MBio 2015;6(3):e00551.

117. Johnson S, Sambol SP, Brazier JS, et al. International typing study of toxin A-negative, toxin B-positive *Clostridium difficile* variants. J Clin Microbiol 2003;41(4):1543–7.

118. Moncrief JS, Zheng L, Neville LM, et al. Genetic characterization of toxin A-negative, toxin B-positive *Clostridium difficile* isolates by PCR. J Clin Microbiol 2000;38(8):3072–5.

119. Samra Z, Talmor S, Bahar J. High prevalence of toxin A-negative toxin B-positive *Clostridium difficile* in hospitalized patients with gastrointestinal disease. Diagn Microbiol Infect Dis 2002;43(3):189–92.

120. Hammond GA, Lyerly DM, Johnson JL. Transcriptional analysis of the toxigenic element of *Clostridium difficile*. Microb Pathog 1997;22(3):143–54.

121. Dupuy B, Govind R, Antunes A, et al. *Clostridium difficile* toxin synthesis is negatively regulated by TcdC. J Med Microbiol 2008;57(Pt 6):685–9.

122. Matamouros S, England P, Dupuy B. *Clostridium difficile* toxin expression is inhibited by the novel regulator TcdC. Mol Microbiol 2007;64(5):1274–88.

123. MacCannell DR, Louie TJ, Gregson DB, et al. Molecular analysis of *Clostridium difficile* PCR ribotype 027 isolates from Eastern and Western Canada. J Clin Microbiol 2006;44(6):2147–52.

124. Warny M, Pepin J, Fang A, et al. Toxin production by an emerging strain of *Clostridium difficile* associated with outbreaks of severe disease in North America and Europe. Lancet 2005;366(9491):1079–84.

125. Barbut F, Decre D, Lalande V, et al. Clinical features of *Clostridium difficile*-associated diarrhoea due to binary toxin (actin-specific ADP-ribosyltransferase)-producing strains. J Med Microbiol 2005;54(Pt 2):181–5.

126. McEllistrem MC, Carman RJ, Gerding DN, et al. A hospital outbreak of *Clostridium difficile* disease associated with isolates carrying binary toxin genes. Clin Infect Dis 2005;40(2):265–72.

127. Rupnik M, Grabnar M, Geric B. Binary toxin producing *Clostridium difficile* strains. Anaerobe 2003;9(6):289–94.

128. Geric B, Carman RJ, Rupnik M, et al. Binary toxin-producing, large clostridial toxin-negative *Clostridium difficile* strains are enterotoxic but do not cause disease in hamsters. J Infect Dis 2006;193(8):1143–50.

129. Joost I, Speck K, Herrmann M, et al. Characterisation of *Clostridium difficile* isolates by *slpA* and *tcdC* gene sequencing. Int J Antimicrob Agents 2009;33(Suppl 1):S13–8.

130. Akerlund T, Persson I, Unemo M, et al. Increased sporulation rate of epidemic *Clostridium difficile* Type 027/NAP1. J Clin Microbiol 2008;46(4):1530–3.

131. Burns DA, Heeg D, Cartman ST, et al. Reconsidering the sporulation characteristics of hypervirulent *Clostridium difficile* BI/NAP1/027. PLoS One 2011;6(9):e24894.

132. Curry SR, Marsh JW, Shutt KA, et al. High frequency of rifampin resistance identified in an epidemic *Clostridium difficile* clone from a large teaching hospital. Clin Infect Dis 2009;48(4):425–9.

133. Chang JY, Antonopoulos DA, Kalra A, et al. Decreased diversity of the fecal Microbiome in recurrent *Clostridium difficile*-associated diarrhea. J Infect Dis 2008;197(3):435–8.

134. Reeves AE, Koenigsknecht MJ, Bergin IL, et al. Suppression of *Clostridium difficile* in the gastrointestinal tracts of germfree mice inoculated with a murine isolate from the family Lachnospiraceae. Infect Immun 2012;80(11):3786–94.
135. Kamiya S, Yamakawa K, Ogura H, et al. Effect of various sodium taurocholate preparations on the recovery of *Clostridium difficile* spores. Microbiol Immunol 1987;31(11):1117–20.
136. Sorg JA, Sonenshein AL. Bile salts and glycine as cogerminants for *Clostridium difficile* spores. J Bacteriol 2008;190(7):2505–12.
137. Sorg JA, Sonenshein AL. Chenodeoxycholate is an inhibitor of *Clostridium difficile* spore germination. J Bacteriol 2009;191(3):1115–7.
138. Koenigsknecht MJ, Theriot CM, Bergin IL, et al. Dynamics and establishment of *Clostridium difficile* infection in the murine gastrointestinal tract. Infect Immun 2015;83(3):934–41.
139. Buffie CG, Bucci V, Stein RR, et al. Precision microbiome reconstitution restores bile acid mediated resistance to *Clostridium difficile*. Nature 2015;517(7533): 205–8.
140. Peterson LR, Olson MM, Shanholtzer CJ, et al. Results of a prospective, 18-month clinical evaluation of culture, cytotoxin testing, and culturette brand (CDT) latex testing in the diagnosis of *Clostridium difficile*-associated diarrhea. Diagn Microbiol Infect Dis 1988;10(2):85–91.
141. Walker RC, Ruane PJ, Rosenblatt JE, et al. Comparison of culture, cytotoxicity assays, and enzyme-linked immunosorbent assay for toxin A and toxin B in the diagnosis of *Clostridium difficile*-related enteric disease. Diagn Microbiol Infect Dis 1986;5(1):61–9.
142. Shanholtzer CJ, Willard KE, Holter JJ, et al. Comparison of the VIDAS *Clostridium difficile* toxin A immunoassay with *C difficile* culture and cytotoxin and latex tests. J Clin Microbiol 1992;30(7):1837–40.
143. Sloan LM, Duresko BJ, Gustafson DR, et al. Comparison of real-time PCR for detection of the *tcdC* gene with four toxin immunoassays and culture in diagnosis of *Clostridium difficile* infection. J Clin Microbiol 2008;46(6):1996–2001.
144. Aichinger E, Schleck CD, Harmsen WS, et al. Nonutility of repeat laboratory testing for detection of *Clostridium difficile* by use of PCR or enzyme immunoassay. J Clin Microbiol 2008;46(11):3795–7.
145. Drees M, Snydman DR, O'Sullivan CE. Repeated enzyme immunoassays have limited utility in diagnosing *Clostridium difficile*. Eur J Clin Microbiol Infect Dis 2008;27(5):397–9.
146. Nemat H, Khan R, Ashraf MS, et al. Diagnostic value of repeated enzyme immunoassays in *Clostridium difficile* infection. Am J Gastroenterol 2009;104(8): 2035–41.
147. Renshaw AA, Stelling JM, Doolittle MH. The lack of value of repeated *Clostridium difficile* cytotoxicity assays. Arch Pathol Lab Med 1996;120(1):49–52.
148. Goldenberg SD, Cliff PR, Smith S, et al. Two-step glutamate dehydrogenase antigen real-time polymerase chain reaction assay for detection of toxigenic *Clostridium difficile*. J Hosp Infect 2010;74(1):48–54.
149. Novak-Weekley SM, Marlowe EM, Miller JM, et al. *Clostridium difficile* testing in the clinical laboratory by use of multiple testing algorithms. J Clin Microbiol 2010;48(3):889–93.
150. Wren MW, Kinson R, Sivapalan M, et al. Detection of *Clostridium difficile* infection: a suggested laboratory diagnostic algorithm. Br J Biomed Sci 2009;66(4): 175–9.

151. Crobach MJ, Dekkers OM, Wilcox MH, et al. European Society of Clinical Microbiology and Infectious Diseases (ESCMID): data review and recommendations for diagnosing *Clostridium difficile*-infection (CDI). Clin Microbiol Infect 2009; 15(12):1053–66.

152. Snell H, Ramos M, Longo S, et al. Performance of the TechLab C. DIFF CHEK-60 enzyme immunoassay (EIA) in combination with the *C difficile* Tox A/B II EIA kit, the Triage *C. difficile* panel immunoassay, and a cytotoxin assay for diagnosis of *Clostridium difficile*-associated diarrhea. J Clin Microbiol 2004;42(10):4863–5.

153. Sunkesula VC, Kundrapu S, Muganda C, et al. Does empirical *Clostridium difficile* infection (CDI) therapy result in false-negative CDI diagnostic test results? Clin Infect Dis 2013;57(4):494–500.

154. Dubberke ER, Han Z, Bobo L, et al. Impact of clinical symptoms on interpretation of diagnostic assays for *Clostridium difficile* infections. J Clin Microbiol 2011;49(8):2887–93.

155. Planche TD, Davies KA, Coen PG, et al. Differences in outcome according to *Clostridium difficile* testing method: a prospective multicentre diagnostic validation study of *C difficile* infection. Lancet Infect Dis 2013;13(11):936–45.

156. Polage CR, Gyorke CE, Kennedy MA, et al. Overdiagnosis of *Clostridium difficile* infection in the molecular test era. JAMA Intern Med 2015;175(11):1792–801.

157. Teasley DG, Gerding DN, Olson MM, et al. Prospective randomised trial of metronidazole versus vancomycin for *Clostridium-difficile*-associated diarrhoea and colitis. Lancet 1983;2(8358):1043–6.

158. Cohen SH, Gerding DN, Johnson S, et al. Clinical practice guidelines for *Clostridium difficile* infection in adults: 2010 update by the society for healthcare epidemiology of America (SHEA) and the Infectious Diseases Society of America (IDSA). Infect Control Hosp Epidemiol 2010;31(5):431–55.

159. Zar FA, Bakkanagari SR, Moorthi KM, et al. A comparison of vancomycin and metronidazole for the treatment of *Clostridium difficile*-associated diarrhea, stratified by disease severity. Clin Infect Dis 2007;45(3):302–7.

160. Johnson S, Louie TJ, Gerding DN, et al. Vancomycin, metronidazole, or tolevamer for *Clostridium difficile* infection: results from two multinational, randomized, controlled trials. Clin Infect Dis 2014;59(3):345–54.

161. Cornely OA, Crook DW, Esposito R, et al. Fidaxomicin versus vancomycin for infection with *Clostridium difficile* in Europe, Canada, and the USA: a double-blind, non-inferiority, randomised controlled trial. Lancet Infect Dis 2012;12(4): 281–9.

162. Cornely OA, Miller MA, Louie TJ, et al. Treatment of first recurrence of *Clostridium difficile* infection: fidaxomicin versus vancomycin. Clin Infect Dis 2012; 55(Suppl 2):S154–61.

163. Louie TJ, Miller MA, Mullane KM, et al. Fidaxomicin versus vancomycin for *Clostridium difficile* infection. N Engl J Med 2011;364(5):422–31.

164. Bauer MP, Kuijper EJ, van Dissel JT, et al. European Society of Clinical Microbiology and Infectious Diseases (ESCMID): treatment guidance document for *Clostridium difficile* infection (CDI). Clin Microbiol Infect 2009;15(12):1067–79.

165. Surawicz CM, Brandt LJ, Binion DG, et al. Guidelines for diagnosis, treatment, and prevention of *Clostridium difficile* infections. Am J Gastroenterol 2013; 108(4):478–98 [quiz: 499].

166. Hamilton MJ, Weingarden AR, Sadowsky MJ, et al. Standardized frozen preparation for transplantation of fecal microbiota for recurrent *Clostridium difficile* infection. Am J Gastroenterol 2012;107(5):761–7.

167. Kelly CR, Ihunnah C, Fischer M, et al. Fecal microbiota transplant for treatment of *Clostridium difficile* infection in immunocompromised patients. Am J Gastroenterol 2014;109(7):1065–71.
168. Kelly CR, Khoruts A, Staley C, et al. Effect of fecal microbiota transplantation on recurrence in multiply recurrent *Clostridium difficile* infection: a randomized trial. Ann Intern Med 2016;165(9):609–16.
169. van Nood E, Vrieze A, Nieuwdorp M, et al. Duodenal infusion of donor feces for recurrent *Clostridium difficile*. N Engl J Med 2013;368(5):407–15.
170. Youngster I, Russell GH, Pindar C, et al. Oral, capsulized, frozen fecal microbiota transplantation for relapsing *Clostridium difficile* infection. JAMA 2014; 312(17):1772–8.
171. Youngster I, Sauk J, Pindar C, et al. Fecal microbiota transplant for relapsing *Clostridium difficile* infection using a frozen inoculum from unrelated donors: a randomized, open-label, controlled pilot study. Clin Infect Dis 2014;58(11): 1515–22.
172. Neal MD, Alverdy JC, Hall DE, et al. Diverting loop ileostomy and colonic lavage: an alternative to total abdominal colectomy for the treatment of severe, complicated *Clostridium difficile* associated disease. Ann Surg 2011;254(3):423–7 [discussion: 427–9].
173. Johnson S, Homann SR, Bettin KM, et al. Treatment of asymptomatic *Clostridium difficile* carriers (fecal excretors) with vancomycin or metronidazole. A randomized, placebo-controlled trial. Ann Intern Med 1992;117(4):297–302.
174. Swale A, Miyajima F, Roberts P, et al. Calprotectin and lactoferrin faecal levels in patients with *Clostridium difficile* infection (CDI): a prospective cohort study. PLoS One 2014;9(8):e106118.
175. D'Haens G, Ferrante M, Vermeire S, et al. Fecal calprotectin is a surrogate marker for endoscopic lesions in inflammatory bowel disease. Inflamm Bowel Dis 2012;18(12):2218–24.
176. Jackson M, Olefson S, Machan JT, et al. A high rate of alternative diagnoses in patients referred for presumed *Clostridium difficile* infection. J Clin Gastroenterol 2016;50(9):742–6.
177. McFarland LV, Surawicz CM, Rubin M, et al. Recurrent *Clostridium difficile* disease: epidemiology and clinical characteristics. Infect Control Hosp Epidemiol 1999;20(1):43–50.
178. Aboudola S, Kotloff KL, Kyne L, et al. *Clostridium difficile* vaccine and serum immunoglobulin G antibody response to toxin A. Infect Immun 2003;71(3): 1608–10.
179. Kelly CP. Immune response to *Clostridium difficile* infection. Eur J Gastroenterol Hepatol 1996;8(11):1048–53.
180. Kyne L, Warny M, Qamar A, et al. Asymptomatic carriage of *Clostridium difficile* and serum levels of IgG antibody against toxin A. N Engl J Med 2000;342(6): 390–7.
181. Kyne L, Warny M, Qamar A, et al. Association between antibody response to toxin A and protection against recurrent *Clostridium difficile* diarrhoea. Lancet 2001;357(9251):189–93.
182. Salcedo J, Keates S, Pothoulakis C, et al. Intravenous immunoglobulin therapy for severe *Clostridium difficile* colitis. Gut 1997;41(3):366–70.
183. Garey KW, Sethi S, Yadav Y, et al. Meta-analysis to assess risk factors for recurrent *Clostridium difficile* infection. J Hosp Infect 2008;70(4):298–304.
184. Sougioultzis S, Kyne L, Drudy D, et al. *Clostridium difficile* toxoid vaccine in recurrent *C difficile*-associated diarrhea. Gastroenterology 2005;128(3):764–70.

185. Lowy I, Molrine DC, Leav BA, et al. Treatment with monoclonal antibodies against *Clostridium difficile* toxins. N Engl J Med 2010;362(3):197–205.

186. Wilcox MH, Gerding DN, Poxton IR, et al. Bezlotoxumab for prevention of recurrent *Clostridium difficile* infection. N Engl J Med 2017;376(4):305–17.

187. Gerding DN, et al. Phase 3 double-blind study of bezlotoxumab (bez) alone and with actoxumab (act) for prevention of recurrent *C. difficile* Infection (rCDI) in patients on standard of care (SoC) antibiotics (MODIFY II). Presented at: Interscience Conference on Antimicrobial Agents and Chemotherapy. San Diego, September 17–21, 2015.

188. Rupnik M, Avesani V, Janc M, et al. A novel toxinotyping scheme and correlation of toxinotypes with serogroups of *Clostridium difficile* isolates. J Clin Microbiol 1998;36(8):2240–7.

189. Lemee L, Dhalluin A, Pestel-Caron M, et al. Multilocus sequence typing analysis of human and animal *Clostridium difficile* isolates of various toxigenic types. J Clin Microbiol 2004;42(6):2609–17.

190. Didelot X, Eyre DW, Cule M, et al. Microevolutionary analysis of *Clostridium difficile* genomes to investigate transmission. Genome Biol 2012;13(12):R118.

191. Songer JG, Trinh HT, Killgore GE, et al. *Clostridium difficile* in retail meat products, USA, 2007. Emerg Infect Dis 2009;15(5):819–21.

192. de Boer E, Zwartkruis-Nahuis A, Heuvelink AE, et al. Prevalence of *Clostridium difficile* in retailed meat in The Netherlands. Int J Food Microbiol 2011;144(3):561–4.

193. Metcalf DS, Costa MC, Dew WM, et al. *Clostridium difficile* in vegetables, Canada. Lett Appl Microbiol 2010;51(5):600–2.

194. Hoffer E, Haechler H, Frei R, et al. Low occurrence of *Clostridium difficile* in fecal samples of healthy calves and pigs at slaughter and in minced meat in Switzerland. J Food Prot 2010;73(5):973–5.

195. Weese JS, Reid-Smith RJ, Avery BP, et al. Detection and characterization of *Clostridium difficile* in retail chicken. Lett Appl Microbiol 2010;50(4):362–5.

196. Jobstl M, Heuberger S, Indra A, et al. *Clostridium difficile* in raw products of animal origin. Int J Food Microbiol 2010;138(1–2):172–5.

197. Houser BA, Soehnlen MK, Wolfgang DR, et al. Prevalence of *Clostridium difficile* toxin genes in the feces of veal calves and incidence of ground veal contamination. Foodborne Pathog Dis 2012;9(1):32–6.

198. Von Abercron SM, Karlsson F, Wigh GT, et al. Low occurrence of *Clostridium difficile* in retail ground meat in Sweden. J Food Prot 2009;72(8):1732–4.

199. Harvey RB, Norman KN, Andrews K, et al. *Clostridium difficile* in poultry and poultry meat. Foodborne Pathog Dis 2011;8(12):1321–3.

200. Harvey RB, Norman KN, Andrews K, et al. *Clostridium difficile* in retail meat and processing plants in Texas. J Vet Diagn Invest 2011;23(4):807–11.

201. Nguyen GC, Kaplan GG, Harris ML, et al. A national survey of the prevalence and impact of *Clostridium difficile* infection among hospitalized inflammatory bowel disease patients. Am J Gastroenterol 2008;103(6):1443–50.

202. Paudel S, Zacharioudakis IM, Zervou FN, et al. Prevalence of *Clostridium difficile* infection among solid organ transplant recipients: a meta-analysis of published studies. PLoS One 2015;10(4):e0124483.

203. Guddati AK, Kumar G, Ahmed S, et al. Incidence and outcomes of *Clostridium difficile*-associated disease in hematopoietic cell transplant recipients. Int J Hematol 2014;99(6):758–65.

204. Lee CH, Steiner T, Petrof EO, et al. Frozen vs fresh fecal microbiota transplantation and clinical resolution of diarrhea in patients with recurrent *Clostridium difficile* infection: a randomized clinical trial. JAMA 2016;315(2):142–9.

Chikungunya Virus

David M. Vu, MD[a],*, Donald Jungkind, PhD[b,1],
Angelle Desiree LaBeaud, MD, MS[a]

KEYWORDS

- Chikungunya virus • Alphavirus • Arbovirus • Togaviridae

KEY POINTS

- Chikungunya is an arboviral infection that causes debilitating arthritis and arthralgia.
- Chikungunya virus has caused explosive epidemics in the past decade, and has spread rapidly from Africa to Asia to the Americas.
- Improved diagnostic testing and surveillance for chikungunya infection is needed to detect and respond to future outbreaks.
- Further investigation into the pathogenesis of chikungunya infection is needed to understand its long-term sequelae, and to develop effective therapies.

MICROBIOLOGY

Chikungunya virus (CHIKV) belongs to the Semliki Forest antigenic group of the genus *Alphaviridae*, which includes other arthritogenic alphaviruses, such as o'nyong-nyong, Ross River, Barmah Forest, and Mayaro viruses.[1,2] Its genome is closely related to that of o'nyong-nyong virus, and consists of a single 11.8-kbp strand of positive sense RNA, which encodes a 2472 amino acid nonstructural and a 1244 amino acid structural polyprotein.[3] The polyproteins give rise to the four nonstructural proteins (nsP1-4) that make up the viral replication machine, and five structural proteins. Each spherical viral particle is approximately 70 nm in diameter and is comprised of a strand of genomic RNA, encapsidated by capsid (C) proteins, surrounded by a host cell–derived lipid bilayer spiked with heterodimers of envelope proteins E1 and E2.[4] The other two structural proteins, 6K and E3, are leader peptides for E1 and E2, respectively, and are not observed in abundance in the mature virion.[4]

Disclosure Statement: The authors have no relevant disclosures.
[a] Department of Pediatrics, Stanford University School of Medicine, 300 Pasteur Drive, G312, Stanford, CA 94305, USA; [b] St. George's University School of Medicine, Grenada, West Indies
[1] Present address: PO Box 4466, Horseshoe Bay, TX 78657.
* Corresponding author.
E-mail address: davidvu@stanford.edu

The envelope proteins, E2 and E1, play important roles in the binding of the virus to the host cell membrane and its subsequent cellular invasion, respectively. Anti-CHIKV antibodies directed against the envelope protein that neutralize the virus in vitro also protect neonatal mice from lethal CHIKV infection in vivo, suggesting that these proteins may be important antigenic lethal targets for development of naturally acquired, or vaccine-elicited protection.[5–7]

EPIDEMIOLOGY

The earliest report of chikungunya fever described an outbreak of a dengue-like illness that occurred in 1952 to 1953, on the Makonde Plateau in the Southern Province of Tanganyika (present day Tanzania).[8] Residents of all ages experienced a febrile illness with rash and arthralgia. However, certain aspects of this outbreak distinguished it from previous reports of dengue fever outbreaks. Most striking was the severity of the arthralgia that "would prevent the sufferer from changing position without help."[8] The local population began to call the disease chikungunya, which is a Makonde (Bantu) term that means "that which bends up," referring to the contorted positions of those who were affected by the sudden and severe onset of arthralgia. Additionally, many individuals affected with the disease continued to experience intermittent joint pains that persisted for months after the acute illness. The attack rate also seemed to be unusually high, often affecting entire households. Between 1952 and 1953, an estimated 60% to 80% of the population in this region developed symptoms of fever, rash, and arthralgia.[8] Attempts to isolate the pathologic agent from symptomatic individuals during the outbreak also diverged from previous experience with dengue virus (DENV): Inoculation of infant mice with serum samples from symptomatic individuals resulted in death of the animals. In contrast, DENV infection is difficult to establish in mice.[9] These data suggested that the cause of the syndrome termed chikungunya indeed was distinct from the cause of dengue fever.

In Africa, CHIKV is transmitted by arboreal Aedes mosquitoes (A furcifer-taylori, A africanus, A luteocephalus, and A neoafricanus) in an enzootic cycle with nonhuman primates as the principle reservoir (**Fig. 1**).[10–12] Between the 1960s and 1990s, incidental human infection led to numerous, small-scale CHIKV outbreaks in countries throughout Central and Southern Africa, and Senegal, Guinea, and Nigeria in Western Africa (reviewed in Ref.[13]). The outbreaks occurred after periods of large rainfall and associated surges in the arboreal Aedes mosquito density. In contrast, CHIKV outbreaks in Southeast Asia occurred in larger cities where Aedes aegypti mosquitoes were implicated as the primary transmission vector. A aegypti mosquitoes require very small amounts of water to lay eggs, and thrive in human urban environments, particularly in areas where residents store water in open containers or cisterns.

In 2004, a large-scale CHIKV epidemic erupted, sweeping down the coast of Kenya into islands on the Indian Ocean (Comoros, Mayotte, Seychelles, Réunion, Madagascar, Sri Lanka, and the Maldives), India, Southeast Asia (Malaysia, Singapore, Thailand), and China.[14] Although CHIKV infection in travelers returning to Europe had been reported previously, autochthonous transmission of CHIKV was observed for the first time in Italy in 2007,[15] and in France in 2009.[16] An important factor that facilitated the rapid expansion of CHIKV infection was a novel single amino acid substitution of alanine for valine at position 226 (A226V) in the E1 envelope protein that enhanced the ability of the Aedes albopictus mosquito to transmit CHIKV to humans.[17] A albopictus is an anthropophilic, peridomestic species of mosquito that

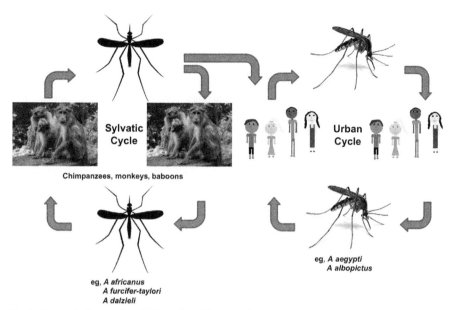

Fig. 1. Transmission cycle of CHIKV in Africa. Nonhuman primates, and possibly other wild animals, serve as reservoirs of the virus. Infected arboreal *Aedes* mosquitoes bite and infect humans. Infected humans, in turn, infect peridomestic *Aedes aegypti*, perpetuating the urban cycle of CHIKV transmission. (*From* Thiboutot MM, Kannan S, Kawalekar OU, et al. Chikungunya: a potentially emerging epidemic? PLoS Negl Trop Dis 2010;4(4):e623.)

has an even greater geographic range than that of its relative, *A aegypti*, and has been implicated as having a major role in the spread of CHIKV epidemics across Asia and to the Americas.

In December 2013, the first cases of locally transmitted CHIKV in the Americas were confirmed in St. Martin,[18] followed rapidly by cases identified throughout the Caribbean and Latin America. By January 2015, CHIKV infection had been identified in 42 countries or territories in the Caribbean, Central America, South America, and North America (local transmission in Florida) with more than a million suspected cases reported, and more than 25,000 laboratory-confirmed.[19]

Although epidemics of febrile arthralgia have been reported in the Americas since the 1700s, these outbreaks previously had been attributed to dengue fever. For example, an epidemic "break-bone fever," which referred to modern-day dengue fever, erupted on the islands of St. Thomas and Santa Cruz in the West Indies from 1827 to 1828. Stedman, who reported this "anomalous disease" called "dandy fever" by local residents, noted that the illness "attacked almost every individual in the town," had "extremely low mortality," and was associated with "pains in the joints for weeks after recovery from the acute stage," which were key differences between the 1827 and 1828 West Indies epidemic and previous descriptions of a "break-bone fever" (referring to modern-day dengue fever). He concluded that "the diseases, though somewhat alike in a few symptoms, are essentially different."[20] Thus, although the 2013 epidemic was the first CHIKV outbreak in the Americas to be confirmed using modern-day virologic methods, historical reports raise questions to whether this truly was the first introduction of CHIKV infection to the Americas.[21]

PATHOGENESIS

CHIKV is known to infect a variety of cell lines in vitro, including Vero cells (from green monkey kidney)[22] and BHK21 baby hamster kidney cells,[23] and various insect cell lines.[24,25] Human cellular tropism was more recently described.[26] Fibroblasts in the dermis, joint capsule, and muscle seem to be the major targets of CHIKV infection in humans.[27] Human epithelial and endothelial cells[26] and muscle progenitors (satellite cells)[28] also have been observed to be infected by CHIKV. Lymphocytes and monocytes seem resistant, yet macrophages seem susceptible to CHIKV infection.[26]

Investigations of disease pathogenesis during human CHIKV infection have been limited, in part, by the lack of relevant and/or accessible models of CHIKV disease. Development of nonhuman primate models of CHIKV infection has been helpful for use in evaluating potential CHIKV vaccines. Rhesus macaques immunized with an investigational CHIKV virus-like particle vaccine were protected against developing viremia after intravenous challenge with 10^{10} PFU of CHIKV, whereas control monkeys that received the mock vaccine developed high levels of viremia after challenge.[29] In a separate study, cynomolgus macaques challenged with a much lower CHIKV inoculum, by either intravenous or intradermal injection, developed viremia, fever, and rash. Viral RNA remained detectable in synovial and muscle tissue for up to 1.5 months after infection, and in lymphoid tissue for up to 3 months.[30] Thus, this model may be useful for studying long-term sequelae of CHIKV infection, such as the prolonged arthralgia experienced by many CHIKV individuals.

Because nonhuman primate models of CHIKV infection are not readily accessible to many investigators, some investigators have developed mouse models to study CHIKV disease. Viral challenge of neonatal wild-type mice results in fatal infection. However, this susceptibility to CHIKV infection wanes quickly and adult wild-type mice are resistant to CHIKV infection. Type I interferon receptor knock-out mice (IFN-α/βR$^{-/-}$) have an impaired type I IFN pathway and, in contrast with adult wild-type mice, develop viremia after viral challenge.[27] Thus, it seems that activation of the type I IFN pathway plays an important role in controlling CHIKV infection.

Mice also have been used to develop models of CHIKV-related arthritis.[31,32] One group of investigators demonstrated that mice injected with CHIKV in the footpad developed leg swelling and weight loss, and had histologic evidence of necrotizing myositis, arthritis, tenosynovitis, and vasculitis.[32] A separate group of investigators also elicited foot swelling in mice injected with CHIKV in the ventral footpad. These mice developed viremia, and histologic examination revealed large mononuclear cell infiltrates in and around synovial membranes, and in muscle tissue. Furthermore, treatment with IFN-α before CHIKV inoculation reduced viremia and prevented manifestations of arthritis,[31] again highlighting the importance of type I IFNs in CHIKV virus control.

CLINICAL MANIFESTATIONS

In contrast to DENV, which can cause asymptomatic infection, most individuals with CHIKV infection are symptomatic.[8] However, chikungunya fever shares many similarities with dengue fever. Sudden onset of high fever is typically the initial symptom reported and can appear within 2 days of infection. A rash sometimes is observed and is typically maculopapular, although bullous rashes have been noted in some infants with CHIKV infection.[33] Both viral infections also are known to cause arthralgia and arthritis. However, the polyarthralgia caused by CHIKV frequently is characterized as debilitating and has been reported to continue well beyond the resolution of fever. For example, a third of travelers to the Caribbean who acquired

CHIKV infection in 2014 while abroad reported persistent joint or muscle pain, or joint swelling at greater than or equal to 9 months after their acute infection.[34] The knees are the most commonly involved joints; however, other large or small joints may be affected. Of note, symmetric involvement of joints is frequently reported.[35] Additional symptoms reported include fatigue, nausea, vomiting, and conjunctivitis. Conspicuously absent among those with CHIKV infection are reports of retro-orbital headache, which are characteristic of dengue fever.[8] Most symptoms resolve within 7 to 10 days; however, many infected individuals have reported protracted arthralgia that has lasted weeks, months, or even years. This long-term burden of disease can be devastating to local economies and represents a significant health cost: CHIKV was responsible for 1386 to 1,081,962 nondiscounted years of life lost in 2005.[36] These values are now significant underestimations of the true health cost burden, given its expanding distribution to the Americas since those estimates were made.

Neurologic complications of acute CHIKV disease were observed with the 2006 outbreak on La Réunion Island, and include encephalitis[37] and Guillain-Barré syndrome.[38] These also were observed during CHIKV outbreaks in India.[39–41] Additional observations of severe manifestations of disease, including myocarditis and hepatitis,[37] have re-energized investigations of CHIKV disease pathogenesis.

CHIKV infection had not been associated with increased risk of mortality before 2006. During the outbreak on La Réunion Island, however, at least 213 people with CHIKV infection died. Investigators estimated that the case-fatality rate was approximately 1:1000, and observed that the fatalities occurred mainly in persons greater than or equal to 75 years of age.[42] During the 2006 outbreak of CHIKV infection in Ahmedabad, India, 18 of the 90 confirmed cases of CHIKV infection were fatal. Fifteen of the 18 deaths occurred in persons 60 years of age and older.[43] Autopsy of fatal cases of CHIKV infection in Colombia revealed evidence of hepatocellular coagulative necrosis, tubulointerstitial nephritis, and acute pericarditis.[44]

DIAGNOSTIC EVALUATION

Good laboratory testing services are important in the diagnosis of suspected CHIKV infections. Chikungunya fever can easily be confused at various stages of the disease with other arboviral infections, such as dengue and Zika virus. The clinical consequences of these three viruses are different, so specific diagnosis is important. Situations where laboratory test confirmation for presence or absence of infection are discussed next.

Testing sporadic cases of suspected arboviral infection can provide early warning that the virus is in the community. This can help public health and medical personnel prevent a possible epidemic. This is especially important if conditions conducive to an epidemic are present, such as during the rainy season when the mosquito population is high, and with open housing conditions that enhance exposure of an immunologically naive population to infection. Diagnosis of a significant number of cases early on to establish cause of an epidemic and the characteristic symptoms enables reliable clinical diagnosis with decreased need for laboratory confirmation if an epidemic occurs. Public health departments may occasionally perform epidemiologic testing for evidence of past CHIKV infection in a community so that the immunologic history and state of susceptibility in a population are determined to better approximate risk for an outbreak.

Focused and random spot testing is important during an epidemic to detect the entrance of a second arbovirus, such as DENV, entering the population during a

CHIKV outbreak. Focused testing is important in cases with serious underlying diseases and in cases with complications or a fatal outcome.

In the postoutbreak period, persons not previously tested for CHIKV should be tested for a recent or past infection as part of the work-up in patients presenting with new chronic arthritic problems including joint pain and swelling. During interepidemic periods, patients presenting with typical CHIKV symptoms should be tested for CHIKV and other arboviruses with similar symptoms.

Three tests for CHIKV are useful in various situations. For diagnostic confirmation of current and recent infection, a molecular test (typically polymerase chain reaction [PCR]) for the virus and an assay for the presence of specific IgM antibody are required. The most frequently needed assay is the CHIKV IgM antibody assay. Molecular testing for the presence of the virus is required in the early stages of disease. Virus is present in the blood at the time symptoms appear and PCR testing provides reliable detection for 5 days thereafter (6 days total). During that time only a molecular test for the virus should be ordered. As IgM production rises, by Days 7 to 9, viremia falls to PCR undetectable levels. During Days 5 to 9 when the viral load is waning and IgM has not reached its peak, it is necessary to order a molecular test for the virus and the IgM antibody assay to maintain good diagnostic sensitivity. After that, only the IgM test is required. After 14 to 21 days both the IgM and IgG test are positive, and the IgM test wanes over several weeks or months, whereas IgG remains for years as a good marker of past infection and immunologic protection, and also as an epidemiologic tool to determine seroprevalence in a population.

Using Grenada as a case study to illustrate the CHIKV diagnostic strategy, during the peak of the 2014 Grenada CHIKV epidemic, 112 samples from typical cases were tested by PCR and the IgM assay independent of the stage of disease. Although all 112 had classic symptoms, only 101 were found to be positive by at least one of these laboratory tests. In the 101 samples, IgM outperformed PCR: 92% were positive by IgM, 17% were positive by PCR, and 9% were positive by both. Reliance on PCR testing only is unlikely to accurately characterize incidence.[45–47]

Commercially available kits are of variable quality.[48] PCR assays with favorable performance characteristics are documented in the literature and becoming commercially available for clinical use in other countries; however, they can only be obtained for research use in the United States. Good immunoassays for CHIKV-specific IgM in patient serum are less reliable and available.[49–51] A partial list of sources for molecular viral assays and IgM assays to document CHIKV infection is given in **Table 1**. These sources can serve as starting points to explore test kit choices and capabilities in what it is hoped will be an expanding menu of kits for clinical testing.

Until reliable Food and Drug Administration–approved kits for molecular detection of virus and CHIKV antibodies are available, only the largest commercial and government reference laboratories should consider routine diagnostic testing for CHIKV. The Centers for Disease Control and Prevention has facilities for testing samples to establish transmission of CHIKV in the United States. Some city and state health departments and other government agencies also have this capability. Specific details related to collection and preserving serum for transportation to and testing at regional or national facilities can be found at: http://www.cdc.gov/chikungunya/hc/diagnostic.html.

If an epidemic should require greater testing capacity, the Centers for Disease Control and Prevention and similar agencies in other countries may implement Emergency Use Authorization for diagnostic tools for CHIKV that could be distributed to qualified clinical laboratories that demonstrate proficiency with the assays by successfully testing verification panels for each assay.

Table 1
Sources for commercially available kits for detection of chikungunya virus and IgM and IgG antibody in serum[a]

Company	Address	Product	Comments
Altona Diagnostics, GmbH	Mörkenstrasse 12 22767 Hamburg, Germany	RealStar Chikungunya RT-PCR Kit	
Liferiver Bio-Tech	9855 Towne Center Drive, San Diego, CA 92121	Chikungunya Virus Real Time RT-PCR Kit	CE approved
Primerdesign, Ltd	York House School Lane, Chandler's Ford, United Kingdom, SO53 4DG	Chikungunya Virus Real Time RT-PCR Kit	Dengue, Zika, and chikungunya virus multiplex kit also available
GenWay Biotech, Inc	6777 Nancy Ridge Drive, San Diego, CA 92121	Real Time RT-PCR Kit IgM μ-capture ELISA IgG capture ELISA	Separate PCR kits formatted for two commonly used PCR instrument types Provides PCR and ELISA assays
Euroimmun AG	Seekamp 31, D-23560 Luebeck, Germany	IgM ELISA IgG ELISA	
IBL Tecan US, Inc	9401 Globe Center Drive, Suite 140, Morrisville, NC 27560	Chikungunya IgM μ-capture ELISA	Laboratory ELISA automation
NovaTec Immundiagnostica, GmbH	Waldstrasse 23 A6, Dietzenbach, 63128, Germany	IgG ELISA and an IgM μ-capture ELISA	

Abbreviations: ELISA, enzyme-linked immunosorbent assay; FDA, Food and Drug Administration; RT, reverse transcriptase.
[a] Partial list of companies providing PCR and ELISA kits for detection of CHIKV or human antibody to the virus. None of these are FDA approved for use as diagnostic tests at this time but are considered in the Research Use Only category. One product is CE approved. These tests may prove to be useful adjuncts to assist in the development of future FDA-approved or validated assays.

If CHIKV infection becomes an annual endemic threat in certain regions, there will be a need for testing capability on a more local basis. It would be ideal to have CHIKV detection as part of a routine test panel and supported by the clinical laboratory testing industry. Encouraging research studies suggest that this will be possible, first for PCR and perhaps later for the IgM assays.[46,51,52]

TREATMENT

There is presently no licensed targeted therapy for acute CHIKV infection. Treatment is primarily supportive care and includes the use of analgesic and anti-inflammatory medication, rehydration, and rest. However, research to identify potential new antiviral therapies, or repurposing of existing compounds for treating CHIKV infection is ongoing (**Table 2**; reviewed in Ref.[53]). For example, chloroquine has in vitro activity against several viruses, and has been found to inhibit CHIKV replication in Vero cells.[54] However, it has

Table 2
Examples of investigational strategies under development for treatment of CHIKV

Therapeutic	Mechanism	Data	
		In Vitro	In Vivo
Chloroquine	Inhibits fusion of CHIKV E1 protein with the endosomal membrane	Inhibited CHIKV infection in Vero A cells[54]	No efficacy in clinical trials in patients infected with CHIKV[58]
siRNA targeting CHIKV genes	Inhibits protein synthesis	Inhibited CHIKV replication in Vero-E6 cells (>90%)[59]	Inhibited CHIKV replication in mice when administered 3 d postinfection[59]
Ribavirin	Inhibits viral genome replication by depleting guanosine triphosphate	Inhibited CHIKV replication in Vero cells Synergistic inhibitory effect in combination with IFN-α2b and doxycycline[60]	Reduced the viral load and inflammation in infected ICR mice when combined with doxycycline[57]
Favipiravir (T-705)	Inhibits viral genome replication	Inhibited CHIKV-induced cytopathic effect in Vero A cells[61]	Reduced mortality of infected AG129 mice and protected from neurologic disease[62]
Monoclonal antibody C9	Binds CHIKV E2 glycoprotein	Neutralized CHIKV pseudovirions in HEK293T cells and CHIKV in Vero cells[63]	100% survival of CHIKV-infected mice when given at 8 or 18 h postinfection[63]

Adapted from Abdelnabi R, Neyts J, Delang L. Towards antivirals against chikungunya virus. Antiviral Res 2015;121:62; with permission.

not been shown to have anti-CHIKV effects in vivo. Compounds that may interfere with viral entry, including phenothiazines[55] and flavaglines,[56] are being investigated as potential therapies. Ribavirin has been shown to have in vitro activity against CHIKV, and synergized with doxycycline to reduce viral load and inflammation in infected mice.[57]

Monoclonal antibodies to the CHIKV E1 and E2 proteins have been used to protect mice and nonhuman primates from developing CHIKV infection after viral challenge.[27,29] However, it is unclear whether passive immunization with monoclonal antibodies or hyperimmune serum can ameliorate symptomatology of CHIKV disease after infection has already been established.

SUMMARY

The past decade has seen explosive viral epidemics, from severe acute respiratory syndrome to Ebola to arboviruses including Zika and CHIKV. For some diseases, the human toll is acutely evident in the form of mortality or acute morbidity. For CHIKV and others, the long-term sequelae from infection are yet ill-defined. The prolonged debilitating arthralgia associated with CHIKV infection has tremendous potential for impacting the global economy, and should be considered when evaluating the human burden of disease and the allocation of resources. There is much still unknown about

CHIKV and the illnesses that it causes. Developing a better understanding of the pathogenesis of CHIKV infection is a priority and forms the basis for developing effective strategies at infection prevention and disease control.

REFERENCES

1. Strauss JH, Strauss EG. The alphaviruses: gene expression, replication, and evolution. Microbiol Rev 1994;58(3):491–562.
2. Lwande OW, Obanda V, Bucht G, et al. Global emergence of alphaviruses that cause arthritis in humans. Infect Ecol Epidemiol 2015;5:29853.
3. Khan AH, Morita K, Parquet Md Mdel C, et al. Complete nucleotide sequence of chikungunya virus and evidence for an internal polyadenylation site. J Gen Virol 2002;83(Pt 12):3075–84.
4. Jose J, Snyder JE, Kuhn RJ. A structural and functional perspective of alphavirus replication and assembly. Future Microbiol 2009;4(7):837–56.
5. Weger-Lucarelli J, Aliota MT, Kamlangdee A, et al. Identifying the role of e2 domains on alphavirus neutralization and protective immune responses. PLoS Negl Trop Dis 2015;9(10):e0004163.
6. Fong RH, Banik SS, Mattia K, et al. Exposure of epitope residues on the outer face of the chikungunya virus envelope trimer determines antibody neutralizing efficacy. J Virol 2014;88(24):14364–79.
7. Smith SA, Silva LA, Fox JM, et al. Isolation and characterization of broad and ultrapotent human monoclonal antibodies with therapeutic activity against chikungunya virus. Cell Host Microbe 2015;18(1):86–95.
8. Robinson MC. An epidemic of virus disease in Southern Province, Tanganyika Territory, in 1952-53. I. Clinical features. Trans R Soc Trop Med Hyg 1955;49(1): 28–32.
9. Ross RW. The Newala epidemic. III. The virus: isolation, pathogenic properties and relationship to the epidemic. J Hyg (Lond) 1956;54(2):177–91.
10. Diallo M, Thonnon J, Traore-Lamizana M, et al. Vectors of chikungunya virus in Senegal: current data and transmission cycles. Am J Trop Med Hyg 1999; 60(2):281–6.
11. McIntosh BM, Paterson HE, McGillivray G, et al. Further studies on the chikungunya outbreak in southern Rhodesia in 1962. I. Mosquitoes, wild primates and birds in relation to the epidemic. Ann Trop Med Parasitol 1964;58:45–51.
12. Paterson HE, McIntosh BM. Further studies on the chikungunya outbreak in southern Rhodesia in 1962. II. Transmission experiments with the *Aedes furcifer-taylori* group of mosquitoes and with a member of the *Anopheles gambiae* complex. Ann Trop Med Parasitol 1964;58:52–5.
13. Powers AM, Logue CH. Changing patterns of chikungunya virus: re-emergence of a zoonotic arbovirus. J Gen Virol 2007;88(Pt 9):2363–77.
14. Kariuki Njenga M, Nderitu L, Ledermann JP, et al. Tracking epidemic chikungunya virus into the Indian Ocean from East Africa. J Gen Virol 2008;89(Pt 11): 2754–60.
15. Rezza G, Nicoletti L, Angelini R, et al. Infection with chikungunya virus in Italy: an outbreak in a temperate region. Lancet 2007;370(9602):1840–6.
16. Grandadam M, Caro V, Plumet S, et al. Chikungunya virus, southeastern France. Emerg Infect Dis 2011;17(5):910–3.
17. Tsetsarkin KA, Vanlandingham DL, McGee CE, et al. A single mutation in chikungunya virus affects vector specificity and epidemic potential. PLoS Pathog 2007; 3(12):e201.

18. Fischer M, Staples JE, Arboviral Diseases Branch, National Center for Emerging and Zoonotic Infectious Diseases, CDC. Notes from the field: chikungunya virus spreads in the Americas - Caribbean and South America, 2013-2014. MMWR Morb Mortal Wkly Rep 2014;63(22):500–1.
19. The Pan American Health Organization. Number of reported cases of chikungunya fever in the Americas, by country or territory 2013-2014 cumulative cases (updated 23 Oct 2015). Number of Reported Cases of Chikungunya Fever in the Americas 2015; 2016. Available at: http://www.paho.org/hq/index.php?option=com_topics&view=readall&cid=5927&Itemid=40931&lang=en. Accessed October 1, 2016.
20. Carey DE. Chikungunya and dengue: a case of mistaken identity? J Hist Med Allied Sci 1971;26(3):243–62.
21. Halstead SB. Reappearance of chikungunya, formerly called dengue, in the Americas. Emerg Infect Dis 2015;21(4):557–61.
22. Higashi N, Matsumoto A, Tabata K, et al. Electron microscope study of development of chikungunya virus in green monkey kidney stable (Vero) cells. Virology 1967;33(1):55–69.
23. Hahon N, Zimmerman WD. Chikungunya virus infection of cell monolayers by cell-to-cell and extracellular transmission. Appl Microbiol 1970;19(2):389–91.
24. Buckley SM, Singh KR, Bhat UK. Small- and large-plaque variants of chikungunya virus in two vertebrate and seven invertebrate cell lines. Acta Virol 1975;19(1):10–8.
25. Cunningham A, Buckley SM, Casals J, et al. Isolation of chikungunya virus contaminating an Aedes albopictus cell line. J Gen Virol 1975;27(1):97–100.
26. Sourisseau M, Schilte C, Casartelli N, et al. Characterization of reemerging chikungunya virus. PLoS Pathog 2007;3(6):e89.
27. Couderc T, Chretien F, Schilte C, et al. A mouse model for chikungunya: young age and inefficient type-I interferon signaling are risk factors for severe disease. PLoS Pathog 2008;4(2):e29.
28. Ozden S, Huerre M, Riviere JP, et al. Human muscle satellite cells as targets of chikungunya virus infection. PLoS One 2007;2(6):e527.
29. Akahata W, Yang ZY, Andersen H, et al. A virus-like particle vaccine for epidemic chikungunya virus protects nonhuman primates against infection. Nat Med 2010;16(3):334–8.
30. Labadie K, Larcher T, Joubert C, et al. Chikungunya disease in nonhuman primates involves long-term viral persistence in macrophages. J Clin Invest 2010;120(3):894–906.
31. Gardner J, Anraku I, Le TT, et al. Chikungunya virus arthritis in adult wild-type mice. J Virol 2010;84(16):8021–32.
32. Morrison TE, Oko L, Montgomery SA, et al. A mouse model of chikungunya virus-induced musculoskeletal inflammatory disease: evidence of arthritis, tenosynovitis, myositis, and persistence. Am J Pathol 2011;178(1):32–40.
33. Robin S, Ramful D, Zettor J, et al. Severe bullous skin lesions associated with chikungunya virus infection in small infants. Eur J Pediatr 2010;169(1):67–72.
34. Zeana C, Kelly P, Heredia W, et al. Post-chikungunya rheumatic disorders in travelers after return from the Caribbean. Travel Med Infect Dis 2016;14(1):21–5.
35. Manimunda SP, Vijayachari P, Uppoor R, et al. Clinical progression of chikungunya fever during acute and chronic arthritic stages and the changes in joint morphology as revealed by imaging. Trans R Soc Trop Med Hyg 2010;104(6):392–9.

36. Labeaud AD, Bashir F, King CH. Measuring the burden of arboviral diseases: the spectrum of morbidity and mortality from four prevalent infections. Popul Health Metr 2011;9(1):1.

37. Lemant J, Boisson V, Winer A, et al. Serious acute chikungunya virus infection requiring intensive care during the Reunion Island outbreak in 2005-2006. Crit Care Med 2008;36(9):2536–41.

38. Wielanek AC, Monredon JD, Amrani ME, et al. Guillain-Barre syndrome complicating a chikungunya virus infection. Neurology 2007;69(22):2105–7.

39. Rampal, Sharda M, Meena H. Neurological complications in chikungunya fever. J Assoc Physicians India 2007;55:765–9.

40. Singh RK, Tiwari S, Mishra VK, et al. Molecular epidemiology of chikungunya virus: mutation in e1 gene region. J Virol Methods 2012;185(2):213–20.

41. Chandak NH, Kashyap RS, Kabra D, et al. Neurological complications of chikungunya virus infection. Neurol India 2009;57(2):177–80.

42. Josseran L, Paquet C, Zehgnoun A, et al. Chikungunya disease outbreak, Reunion Island. Emerg Infect Dis 2006;12(12):1994–5.

43. Tandale BV, Sathe PS, Arankalle VA, et al. Systemic involvements and fatalities during chikungunya epidemic in India, 2006. J Clin Virol 2009;46(2):145–9.

44. Mercado M, Acosta-Reyes J, Parra E, et al. Clinical and histopathological features of fatal cases with dengue and chikungunya virus co-infection in Colombia, 2014 to 2015. Euro Surveill 2016. [Epub ahead of print].

45. Jungkind D, Myers TE, Simmons M, et al. Establishment of laboratory testing capability for chikungunya virus in Grenada, West Indies. Presented at the Caribbean Public Health Agency: 60th Annual Scientific Meeting. The University of the West Indies, June 20-24, 2015.

46. Simmons M, Myers T, Guevara C, et al. Development and validation of a quantitative, one-step, multiplex, real-time reverse transcriptase PCR assay for detection of dengue and chikungunya viruses. J Clin Microbiol 2016;54(7):1766–73.

47. Macpherson CNL, Noel T, Jungkind D, et al. Clinical, molecular and serological outcomes of the chikungunya outbreak in Grenada. Presented at the Caribbean Public Health Agency: 60th Annual Scientific Meeting. The University of the West Indies. 2015.

48. Soh LT, Squires RC, Tan LK, et al. External quality assessment of dengue and chikungunya diagnostics in the Asia Pacific region, 2015. Western Pac Surveill Response J 2016;7(2):26–34.

49. Prat CM, Flusin O, Panella A, et al. Evaluation of commercially available serologic diagnostic tests for chikungunya virus. Emerg Infect Dis 2014;20(12):2129–32.

50. Kam YW, Pok KY, Eng KE, et al. Sero-prevalence and cross-reactivity of chikungunya virus specific anti-e2ep3 antibodies in arbovirus-infected patients. PLoS Negl Trop Dis 2015;9(1):e3445.

51. Parashar D, Paingankar MS, Sudeep AB, et al. Assessment of qPCR, nested RT-PCR and ELISA techniques in diagnosis of chikungunya. Curr Sci 2014;107(12):2011–3.

52. Macpherson C, Noel T, Fields P, et al. Clinical and serological insights from the Asian lineage chikungunya outbreak in Grenada, 2014: an observational study. Am J Trop Med Hyg 2016;95(4):890–3.

53. Abdelnabi R, Neyts J, Delang L. Towards antivirals against chikungunya virus. Antiviral Res 2015;121:59–68.

54. Khan M, Santhosh SR, Tiwari M, et al. Assessment of in vitro prophylactic and therapeutic efficacy of chloroquine against chikungunya virus in Vero cells. J Med Virol 2010;82(5):817–24.

55. Pohjala L, Utt A, Varjak M, et al. Inhibitors of alphavirus entry and replication identified with a stable chikungunya replicon cell line and virus-based assays. PLoS One 2011;6(12):e28923.
56. Wintachai P, Thuaud F, Basmadjian C, et al. Assessment of flavaglines as potential chikungunya virus entry inhibitors. Microbiol Immunol 2015;59(3):129–41.
57. Rothan HA, Bahrani H, Mohamed Z, et al. A combination of doxycycline and ribavirin alleviated chikungunya infection. PLoS One 2015;10(5):e0126360.
58. Chopra A, Saluja M, Venugopalan A. Effectiveness of chloroquine and inflammatory cytokine response in patients with early persistent musculoskeletal pain and arthritis following chikungunya virus infection. Arthritis Rheumatol 2014;66(2): 319–26.
59. Parashar D, Paingankar MS, Kumar S, et al. Administration of e2 and ns1 siRNAs inhibit chikungunya virus replication in vitro and protects mice infected with the virus. PLoS Negl Trop Dis 2013;7(9):e2405.
60. Briolant S, Garin D, Scaramozzino N, et al. In vitro inhibition of chikungunya and Semliki forest viruses replication by antiviral compounds: synergistic effect of interferon-alpha and ribavirin combination. Antiviral Res 2004;61(2):111–7.
61. Jadav SS, Sinha BN, Hilgenfeld R, et al. Thiazolidone derivatives as inhibitors of chikungunya virus. Eur J Med Chem 2015;89:172–8.
62. Delang L, Segura Guerrero N, Tas A, et al. Mutations in the chikungunya virus non-structural proteins cause resistance to favipiravir (T-705), a broad-spectrum antiviral. J Antimicrob Chemother 2014;69(10):2770–84.
63. Selvarajah S, Sexton NR, Kahle KM, et al. A neutralizing monoclonal antibody targeting the acid-sensitive region in chikungunya virus e2 protects from disease. PLoS Negl Trop Dis 2013;7(9):e2423.

Rickettsiae as Emerging Infectious Agents

Rong Fang, MD, PhD[a], Lucas S. Blanton, MD[b], David H. Walker, MD[c],*

KEYWORDS

- Rickettsiae • Taxonomy • Rickettsioses • Pathogenesis • Transmission
- Epidemiology • Clinical manifestations • Laboratory diagnosis

KEY POINTS

- Since first discovered by Howard Ricketts in 1906, 27 species of rickettsiae have emerged, of which at least 17 are pathogenic to humans.
- Pathogenic rickettsiae are introduced into a person's skin in association with arthropod vectors, spread via lymphatics to draining lymph nodes, and disseminate hematogenously to infect microvascular endothelial cells, which leads to severe illness.
- Clinical manifestations of rickettsial diseases usually include fever, headache, and rash. Severe cases develop interstitial pneumonia, meningoencephalitis, and multiorgan failure.
- Although serology confirms the diagnosis, detection of rickettsial antigen by immunohistochemistry or DNA by polymerase chain reaction in skin samples serves as a reliable assay for early diagnosis.
- Tetracyclines are the drug class of choice for the treatment of all spotted fever group and typhus group rickettsioses, with doxycycline being the preferred agent.

Rickettsia are obligately intracellular, small (0.3–0.5×0.8–2.0 μm) bacilli with a gram-negative cell wall that has typical bilayer inner and outer membranes separated by a periplasmic layer. Rickettsiae reside free in the cytosol where they replicate by binary fission. Owing to reductive evolution, rickettsiae have small genomes (1.1–1.5 Mb), reflecting the ability of these organisms to survive without some biosynthetic pathways by obtaining these molecules from the host cell.[1] This article presents the history, taxonomy, and microbiology of these intracellular bacteria. It also includes the

Disclosure: The authors have nothing to disclose.
[a] Department of Pathology, The University of Texas Medical Branch at Galveston, 301 University Boulevard, Galveston, TX 77555-0609, USA; [b] Infectious Diseases, Department of Internal Medicine, The University of Texas Medical Branch at Galveston, 301 University Boulevard, Galveston, TX 77555-0435, USA; [c] Department of Pathology, Center for Biodefense and Emerging Infectious Diseases, The University of Texas Medical Branch, 301 University Boulevard, Keiller Building, Galveston, TX 77555-0609, USA
* Corresponding author.
E-mail address: dwalker@utmb.edu

pathogenesis, transmission, clinical manifestations, and laboratory diagnosis of rickettsial diseases.

DISCOVERY OF RICKETTSIAL SPECIES

In the sense of discovery, all infectious agents have been identified since the demonstration in 1876 that *Bacillus anthracis* causes anthrax. The first discovery of a *Rickettsia* was achieved by Howard Ricketts in the Bitterroot Valley of Montana in 1906 when he isolated the organisms from the blood of patients by inoculation of guinea pigs, which developed a febrile illness with distinctive scrotal swelling and hemorrhagic necrosis.[2] He also visualized the organisms and detected them in ticks, a model elucidation of an emerging infectious disease.[3] Von Prowazek and da Rochalima in Europe and Ricketts in Mexico identified the causative agent of louse-borne typhus by feeding clean lice on infected patients, observing the development of rickettsial infection in the louse gut, infecting monkeys, and observing the organisms microscopically.[4] This scientific tour de force resulted in the deaths of the investigators from infection with the agent named in their honor, *Rickettsia prowazekii*.

Each subsequent discovery began as a cluster of cases, such as in an apartment building in New York City (*Rickettsia akari*)[5,6]; application of archaic serologic methods (Weil-Felix *Proteus vulgaris* OX-2 and OX-19 strains agglutination) in patients with unknown diseases in Japan and on Flinders Island, Australia (leading to isolation of *Rickettsia japonica*[7] and *Rickettsia honei*,[8] respectively); molecular studies of old isolates (*Rickettsia massiliae*) or patient specimens (*Rickettsia parkeri* and *Candidatus* Rickettsia philippii)[9,10]; or investigation of unusual clinical manifestations, such as lymphangitis in *Rickettsia sibirica* mongolotimonae strain infections[11] and afebrile cervical lymphadenopathy and scalp ulcer in *Rickettsia slovaca* infections.[12] At present, polymerase chain reaction (PCR) studies are leading to the detection of DNA sequences of *Rickettsia* for which a causal role is proposed. Only time, rickettsial isolates from human specimens, detection of a specific immune response, and pursuit of fulfilling Koch postulates will reveal which are truly additional emerging rickettsial diseases.

TAXONOMY

The genus *Rickettsia* comprises an ever-increasing number of named species and agents detected by molecular methods for which taxonomic names have been proposed. Because of their historic association with human diseases and arthropod vectors, scientists have focused on investigation of human diseases and potential vectors such as ticks, mites, fleas, and lice that transmit rickettsiae during feeding in their saliva or through passing *Rickettsia*-infected feces. However, molecular methods have fostered broader searches and discovery of rickettsiae in other sources, such as herbivorous insects, leeches, and amoebas.[13] Phylogenetically these organisms are basal, more closely related to the common ancestor of the genus.

The *List of Prokaryotic Names with Standing in Nomenclature* (Available at: http://www.bacterio.net/. Accessed March 9, 2017) contains 27 species that currently are considered members of the genus *Rickettsia*, of which there is evidence that at least 17 are capable of infecting humans (**Table 1**). Some, such as *Rickettsia peacockii* and *Rickettsia buchneri*, are symbionts of ticks and very unlikely to cause human infections.[14,15] Others, such as *R parkeri*, *R slovaca*, and *R massiliae*, which were in the past considered to be nonpathogenic, are now recognized as agents of human disease.[9,12,16] Other cultivated organisms that have not been formally proposed as unique species, such as strain 364D (proposed name *R philippii*) and *Rickettsia amblyommatis*, are directly and indirectly associated with human infections.[10,17,18]

Table 1
Named organisms of the genus *Rickettsia* and rickettsial diseases

Organism	Group	Disease
Rickettsia rickettsii	SFG	Rocky Mountain spotted fever
Rickettsia prowazekii	Typhus	Epidemic louse-borne typhus
Rickettsia conorii	SFG	Mediterranean spotted fever
Rickettsia typhi	Typhus	Murine typhus
Rickettsia sibirica	SFG	Siberian tick typhus
Rickettsia australis	Transitional	Queensland tick typhus
Rickettsia akari	Transitional	Rickettsialpox
Rickettsia slovaca	SFG	Tick-borne lymphadenopathy
Rickettsia parkeri	SFG	Maculatum disease
Rickettsia japonica	SFG	Japanese spotted fever
Rickettsia honei	SFG	Flinders Island spotted fever
Rickettsia africae	SFG	African tick bite fever
Rickettsia massiliae	SFG	Unnamed spotted fever
Rickettsia aeschlimannii	SFG	Unnamed
Rickettsia heilongjiangensis	SFG	Far Eastern spotted fever
Rickettsia monacensis	SFG	Unnamed
Rickettsia helvetica	SFG	Unnamed
Rickettsia felis	Transitional	Flea-borne spotted fever
Rickettsia raoultii	SFG	
Rickettsia asiatica	SFG	
Rickettsia bellii	Ancestral	
Rickettsia buchneri	SFG	
Rickettsia canadensis	Ancestral	
Rickettsia hoogstraalii	Transitional	
Rickettsia montanensis	SFG	
Rickettsia peacockii	SFG	
Rickettsia rhipicephali	SFG	
Rickettsia tamurae	SFG	
Rickettsia amblyommatis	SFG	Unnamed

Abbreviation: SFG, spotted fever group.

The criteria that are used for justifying that an organism represents a unique *Rickettsia* species are based on percentage of genetic divergence for a set of genes.[19] The level of genetic difference according to these criteria is substantially less than for other bacterial genera.[20,21] For this reason, there is a larger number of species names of *Rickettsia* than there is for the same level of genetic diversity of other bacterial genera, including those of other obligately intracellular bacteria, *Ehrlichia* and *Orientia*. It is unclear how clinically or scientifically useful it is to designate so many strains as individual species.

The phylogeny of *Rickettsia* shows the basal ancestral group, which includes *Rickettsia bellii*, *Rickettsia canadensis*, and very likely an enormous number of uncharacterized species, and the classic spotted fever and typhus groups. The name transitional group has been proposed for organisms that are between the last 2 clades.[22]

PATHOGENESIS AND TRANSMISSION

Pathogenic rickettsiae introduced into a person's skin infect cutaneous phagocytic cells, are likely transported via lymphatic vessels to the draining lymph nodes where they replicate and subsequently enter the bloodstream, are disseminated hematogenously, and infect microvascular endothelial cells. There they initiate pathogenic events leading to increased vascular permeability, rash, and in severe illness interstitial pneumonia, meningoencephalitis, and multiorgan failure.[23]

Transmission of spotted fever group (SFG) rickettsiae occurs during a tick's feeding on the skin. The proportion of ticks that carry rickettsiae varies from a very small fraction (as low as 1 per 2000 ticks) of *Dermacentor variabilis*, *Dermacentor andersoni*, *Amblyomma sculptum*, and *Amblyomma aureolatum* ticks infected with highly pathogenic *Rickettsia rickettsii*[24–27] to 50% or more of *Amblyomma variegatum* and *Amblyomma hebraeum* ticks infected with the mildly pathogenic *Rickettsia africae*.[28] The tick probes the skin, inserts its mouthparts, which cut the epidermis and dermis, creating a small pool of blood into which the hypostome is inserted, and through which blood is ingested and saliva containing anticoagulants, anesthetic, host defense–inhibiting molecules, and rickettsiae is injected. *R akari* is transmitted similarly by feeding gamasid mites, *Liponyssoides sanguineus*.[29]

R prowazekii and *Rickettsia typhi* are transmitted in the feces of human body lice and fleas, respectively, which are deposited on the skin during their taking of a blood meal. The rickettsiae-containing insect feces are presumably scratched into the skin at the site of the wound of the louse or flea bite, or are rubbed onto mucous membranes, such as the conjunctivae.[30,31] *R prowazekii* has also been found in flying squirrels (*Glaucomys volans*) and their flea and louse ectoparasites in the eastern United States.[32] Most likely human infections associated with flying squirrels are transmitted by the flying squirrels' fleas (*Orchopeas howardii*), which also feed on humans.[33] The discovery of *R prowazekii* in ticks in Ethiopia and Mexico suggests that ticks such as *Amblyomma imitator* may transmit these rickettsiae during feeding, as occurs with SFG rickettsiae.[34,35]

EPIDEMIOLOGY AND CLINICAL MANIFESTATIONS
Spotted Fever Group Rickettsioses

Rocky Mountain spotted fever (RMSF), caused by *R rickettsii*, is the most severe rickettsiosis, with untreated and treated case fatality rates of ~23% and 4%, respectively.[23] In the United States it is classically transmitted by *D andersoni* and *D variabilis* ticks and has more recently been implicated in outbreaks involving *Rhipicephalus sanguineus* in Arizona.[36] RMSF also occurs in Central and South America (**Table 2**), where it is transmitted by bites of *Amblyomma* spp. and *Rh sanguineus*.[23] Illness is characterized by fever with accompanying headache and myalgias. Gastrointestinal symptoms (eg, nausea, vomiting, and abdominal pain) are frequently reported[37] and, at times, have been mistaken for an acute surgical abdomen.[38] Rash typically starts 3 to 5 days after the onset of illness (49% of patients have rash during the first 3 days and 90% have rash at some point during the course). It usually begins as macules on the wrists and ankles before spreading proximally to the trunk. Involvement of the hands and soles is considered characteristic (occurs in 36%–82%) but is a late finding.[37] Cutaneous necrosis and gangrene occur in 4%.[39,40]

Most SFG rickettsioses are associated with an inoculation eschar at the site of previous tick attachment and have a variable range of clinical severity. One of the most widely distributed SFG rickettsiae, and the next most severe, is *Rickettsia conorii*, which is the causative agent of Mediterranean spotted fever (MSF). The organism is

Table 2
Clinical and epidemiologic features of rickettsial diseases

Severity	Disease	Organism	Distribution	Vector	Rash (%)	Eschar (%)
+++++	Rocky Mountain spotted fever	R rickettsii	Americas	Tick	90	<1
++++	Typhus	R prowazekii	South America, Africa, Eurasia	Body louse, ectoparasites of flying squirrels	80	None
+++	Mediterranean spotted fever	R conorii	Europe, Africa, Asia	Tick	97	50
+++	Murine typhus	R typhi	Worldwide	Flea	60	None
++	Siberian tick typhus	R sibirica	Eurasia, Africa	Tick	95	100
++	Japanese spotted fever	R japonica	Japan, eastern Asia	Tick	100	94
++	Flinders Island spotted fever	R honei	Australia, Asia	Tick	76	42
++	Far Eastern spotted fever	R heilongjiangensis	Eastern Asia	Tick	92	92
++	Queensland tick typhus	R australis	Eastern Australia	Tick	95	65
++	African tick bite fever	R africae	Sub-Saharan Africa	Tick	50	90
++	Maculatum disease	R parkeri	Americas	Tick	88	94
+ᵃ	Rickettsialpox	R akari	North America, Eurasia	Mouse mite	100	90
+	Flea-borne spotted fever	R felis	Worldwide	Flea	75	13
+	Tick-borne lymphadenopathy	R slovaca	Europe, Asia	Tick	5	100
+ᵇ	Unnamed spotted fever	R massiliae	South America, Europe	Tick	75	75
+ᵇ	Unnamed spotted fever	Candidatus R philippii	United States	Tick	14	100
+ᵇ	Unnamed spotted fever	R aeschlimannii	Africa	Tick	80	60
+ᵇ	Unnamed spotted fever	R monacensis	Europe	Tick	67	33
+ᵇ,ᶜ	Unnamed spotted fever	R helvetica	Europe	Tick	None	13
+/−ᶜ	Asymptomatic or mild illness with seroconversion	R amblyommatis	Americas	Tick	Probably few	None

ᵃ R felis has been identified from blood, eschar, and cerebrospinal fluid specimens by polymerase chain reaction in patients with febrile illness, but the detection of R felis DNA from the blood and skin of asymptomatic humans causes some ambiguity with regard to its pathogenic nature.
ᵇ Clinical data based on a limited number of patients reported in the literature.
ᶜ Implicated as a cause of asymptomatic infection or self-limited illness with subsequent seroconversion.

transmitted by *Rh sanguineus*, and disease occurs throughout southern Europe, northern Africa, the Middle East, and central Asia.[41] Manifestations are similar to RMSF with the addition of an eschar.[42] One of the less severe, but frequently occurring, rickettsial illnesses in travelers to sub-Saharan Africa is African tick bite fever. Because of the frequency of the causative agent, *R africae*, within *Amblyomma* ticks, and the aggressive nature of these ticks, patients often have multiple eschars, which indicate multiple inoculations.[28] In the Americas, a phylogenetically related organism, *R parkeri*, causes a mild eschar-associated rickettsiosis.[9,43] Both of these diseases are accompanied by constitutional symptoms such as fever, headache, and myalgias. Other manifestations include regional lymphadenopathy at the site of the eschar's draining lymph node, diffuse maculopapular rash in some patients, and a sparse vesiculopapular rash in others. Half of patients have no rash. No death has ever been attributed to infection with *R africae* or *R parkeri*.

Tick-borne lymphadenopathy is another SFG rickettsiosis that is slightly different than the aforementioned syndromes. The illness is caused by *R slovaca*, *Rickettsia raoultii*, and other proposed SFG species in Europe and Asia.[41] It is characterized by an inoculation eschar on the head or neck, surrounding alopecia, and regional lymphadenopathy. Fever and rash seldom occur.[44]

Typhus Group Rickettsioses

Louse-borne typhus occurs in epidemics when conditions of war, extreme cold, and poverty promote the proliferation of the body louse (*Pediculus humanus corporis*). Historically, typhus has ravaged armies, prisons, and refugee camps, and has helped shape the outcomes of wars.[30] Although it is often forgotten as the cause of a serious illness, it has been implicated in recent decades in large outbreaks, continues to have an endemic focus in the Peruvian Andes, and has recently been implicated in a youth rehabilitation center in western Rwanda.[45] Unique to typhus is the ability for humans to act as a latent reservoir for *R prowazekii*. When afflicted, and successfully recovered, a latent human infection (perhaps associated with advancing age, alcoholism, or physical stress) can recrudesce and become rickettsemic. If this occurs during a situation of cold, crowded, and body louse–infested conditions among a susceptible population, an epidemic may occur.[30] Illness is characterized by a prodrome of malaise followed by abrupt onset of fever, headache, chills, and myalgias. Rash is macular and usually starts in the axilla or on the trunk before spreading to the extremities. Although the presence of rash was almost universally reported in early descriptions of typhus for which this manifestation was a diagnostic criterion, rash has been noted to occur in 25% to 38% of patients during more recent outbreaks.[46,47] These later descriptions are from Africa, where rash may be difficult to detect in darkly pigmented individuals. Without appropriate antibiotics, death occurs in 13% of patients.[4] The manifestations of recrudescent typhus (Brill-Zinsser disease) are similar to those of nonfatal primary infection.[48] As mentioned previously, a sylvatic cycle of *R prowazekii* transmission involving flying squirrels and their ectoparasites is associated with sporadic cases of typhus in the eastern United States.[49] Flying squirrel–associated typhus is less severe and has had no reported fatalities.

Murine typhus is known to be endemic to tropical and subtropical seaboard regions where the primary reservoir (*Rattus* spp) and flea vector (*Xenopsylla cheopis*) come into close contact with humans, especially in urban environments. In the United States, the disease is endemic in Texas and southern California, where opossums and cat fleas (*Ctenocephalides felis*) have been associated with a suburban cycle of transmission.[31] Generally considered mild, many cases are undiagnosed, and therefore murine typhus is likely vastly under-recognized. As with the aforementioned rickettsioses, fever, headache, and myalgias are characteristic.[50] The incidence of rash is variable, and has been reported in as few as 20% of darkly pigmented individuals and as many as 80% with lightly pigmented skin.[51] In a review of 10 large case series, which included a total of 841 patients, rash was described in 59%.[52] When present, the rash is usually macular or maculopapular. It is usually distributed over the trunk, may occur over the extremities, and is seldom noted on the palms and soles. Death has been reported in up to 4% of patients ill enough to be hospitalized.[50]

Transitional Group Rickettsioses

Queensland tick typhus occurs in eastern Australia, where *Ixodes* spp ticks transmit *Rickettsia australis*. The disease is similar to SFG rickettsioses and is often associated with an eschar.[53] *Rickettsia felis* is transmitted by *C felis*, and, because of the ubiquitous nature of these fleas, disease has been reported throughout the world.[54] Rickettsialpox, caused by *R akari*, is characterized by a primary papule at the site of vector mite feeding that becomes vesicular and eventually forms an eschar. After a few days of illness, a papular rash erupts. In many patients, these papules form vesicles that evolve into multiple small crusts similar to the primary lesion.[55,56] The disease was originally described in New York City,[5] and is primarily an urban disease of the northeastern United States.

LABORATORY DIAGNOSIS OF RICKETTSIAL DISEASES

The clinical diagnosis of a rickettsial infection relies on the patient's symptoms (such as fever, rash and headache), history of possible exposure to infected arthropods or travel to an endemic area, and supporting data from laboratory diagnostic assays. However, because of the limitations of current laboratory diagnostic assays for rickettsial diseases, prompt empiric therapy should not be withheld if such an infection is suspected. Next, this article reviews the diagnostic assays of rickettsial diseases in the clinical laboratory, including their critical features, limitations, and needs for the future.

According to the samples collected and time of onset of clinical symptoms, current laboratory diagnostic assays of rickettsial diseases include immunohistochemical analysis, molecular detection, isolation and culture of pathogens, and serology (**Fig. 1**).

Detection of Rickettsial Antigen by Immunohistochemical Staining

Because rickettsial infections often present with rash or eschar, skin biopsy samples from these lesions are particularly valuable for detection of rickettsial antigen during the acute stage of illness before any empiric antimicrobial treatment. Eschar and cutaneous rash biopsy specimens are first formalin fixed and paraffin embedded (FFPE). Immunohistochemical staining can show rickettsiae that often cause an eschar, such as *R conorii*, *R africae*, *R akari*, and *R parkeri*, in these cutaneous biopsy samples by using antibodies directed or cross reactive against these rickettsial species.[9,57–60] This approach has the ability to reliably yield a diagnosis during the acute stage of rickettsial infection. In patients with RMSF, skin biopsy of the rash has a reported sensitivity and specificity of 70% and 100%, respectively.[61] This technique can be used to detect other members of the SFG as well as those of the typhus group.[57,58] In addition, this technique can serve as a confirmatory assay for autopsy specimens, including those from the skin, liver, spleen, lung, heart, kidney, and brain.[62,63] However, detection of rickettsial antigen often fails by this technique if the cutaneous samples are collected after 48 hours or longer of antimicrobial administration.[64]

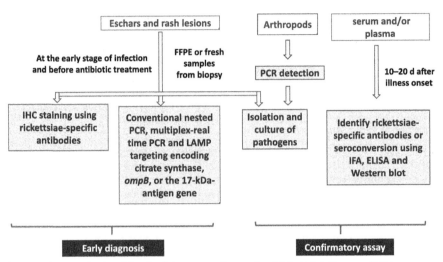

Fig. 1. A diagnostic algorithm for laboratory diagnosis of rickettsial diseases. ELISA, enzyme-linked immunosorbent assay; FFPE, formalin-fixed, paraffin-embedded; IFA, immunofluorescence assay; IHC staining, immunohistochemical staining; LAMP, loop mediated isothermal amplification; OmpB, outer membrane protein B; PCR, polymerase chain reaction.

Molecular Genetic Approaches for Diagnosis

Detection of nucleic acid molecules of rickettsiae in tissue samples using molecular genetic approaches, such as PCR, provides a rapid and reliable diagnostic test in the acute phase of rickettsial infections. Both blood and skin tissue samples can be used for molecular diagnostic assays in clinics. Because of the endothelial tropism of these intracellular bacteria, molecular genetic approaches often achieve much higher sensitivity and specificity in infected skin samples compared with whole blood. Skin biopsy specimens, eschar swabs, and FFPE biopsy specimens have been reported to be used for isolation of DNA followed by amplification of rickettsial gene fragments.[65–68] In contrast, detection of rickettsial DNA in the blood samples often has poor sensitivity,[69,70] except in the late phase of fatal cases. Data from laboratory animal models show that testing of skin samples from sites of rickettsial proliferation can provide definitive molecular diagnosis of up to 60% to 70% of tick-borne SFG rickettsial infections during the acute stage of illness.[71] Conventional, nested, real-time PCR and loop-mediated isothermal amplification assay have been reported as molecular diagnostic tools for rickettsial infections.[72–74] Screening for the presence or absence of rickettsial DNA within a sample can be achieved initially by using genus-specific primers designed to amplify conserved portions of genes encoding citrate synthase, *ompB*, or the 17-kDa antigen gene.[75–77] If a sample screening assay detects target DNA, further analysis using primers to amplify *ompA*, common to the SFG, can help distinguish between an SFG and a typhus group infection. Depending on the targeted genes, molecular diagnostic tools can identify the rickettsial pathogens at either genus-specific and/or species-specific levels, although this does not lead to a difference in the therapeutic interventions. In addition, PCR followed by gene sequencing also provides a species-specific diagnostic result. Recently, multiplex real-time PCR showed greater sensitivity than nested PCR assays in FFPE tissues and provides an effective method to specifically identify cases of RMSF, rickettsialpox, and *R parkeri* rickettsiosis by using skin biopsy specimens.[66] A novel Rick PCR system significantly improved the sensitivity of the PCR test for *R japonica* in peripheral blood samples, and it was close to the sensitivity of conventional PCR using skin samples.[69]

An inexpensive alternative method to sequencing for identification of the rickettsial species is restriction fragment length polymorphism analysis, which can be performed using products amplified from the aforementioned genes. The differentiation of rickettsiae can be achieved by using the endonuclease *AluI* for citrate synthase[77,78] and the 17-kDa antigen gene PCR products.[79] Digestion of an *ompB* PCR product using *RsaI* enables differentiation of several SFG rickettsiae.[78] In addition, a primer set that amplifies a portion of the *ompA* gene digested with a combination of endonucleases (*RsaI*, *PstI*, *AluI*, *XbaI*, and *AvaII*) can identify most of the recognized SFG rickettsiae.[80,81] The use of molecular techniques in recent years has greatly enhanced the sensitivity and specificity of the diagnosis of rickettsial diseases.

Isolation and Culture

For diagnosis of infectious diseases caused by a known pathogen, isolation of the specific micro-organisms is one of the most traditional approaches. Laboratory isolation of rickettsiae can also serve as one of the most confirmatory assays for diagnosis of rickettsial diseases. Blood, skin, and arthropod samples from a suspected patient can be used for isolation of these organisms by cell culture. However, laboratory isolation and culture of rickettsiae from clinical samples for diagnosis require technical expertise and specialized facilities. Because a small amount of aerosolized rickettsiae can cause illness, isolation of rickettsiae requires performance in a biosafety level-3 laboratory. Rickettsiae are obligately intracellular organisms and require appropriate host cells for cultivation. Culture of these organisms may also take a significant amount of time for growth to be detected compared with more typical bacteria. Samples such as skin or arthropods are often not sterile and need to be treated or processed for further culture. These challenges limit isolation as a method for diagnosis in acute infections. Shell vial culture followed by real-time PCR has been applied in the research laboratory to detection of *R conorii*, *R typhi*, and *R felis*.[82–84]

Serology

Detection of antibodies in the serum or plasma of patients infected with rickettsiae is a gold-standard assay for confirming the diagnosis of rickettsial infections. Rickettsial antigen-specific antibodies can be detected by enzyme-linked immunosorbent assay (ELISA), indirect immunofluorescence assay (IFA), and Western blot.[64,85,86] The patient antibody response lags behind the onset of clinical illness. As a patient's illness progresses, a detectable antibody response follows, usually after 7 to 10 days but in some cases after 2 to 3 weeks. The immunoglobulin (Ig) M and IgG responses occur nearly simultaneously in patients with RMSF. Levels of antibodies of both isotypes increase during the second week of illness.[85] Because the appearance of IgM does not occur sooner, and IgM antibodies cross react with nonrickettsial antigens more often than the IgG isotype, testing for IgM does not offer greater sensitivity or specificity during early illness.

The gold-standard serologic method for diagnosis of RMSF is the IFA. This method uses a fluorescein-labeled conjugate to detect serum antibodies bound to antigen (*R rickettsii*–infected cells) fixed on a slide. The performance of IFA with regard to sensitivity and specificity has greatly surpassed that of older methods, such as Weil-Felix, latex agglutination, and complement fixation.[87] The test is available commercially and is also available through state public health laboratories. The sensitivity of IFA 2 weeks after the onset of illness is 94% to 100%.[64] Because IFA predictably fails to detect antibodies during the acute phase of illness, paired sera should be obtained during the acute illness and after convalescence. Seroconversion or a 4-fold increase from acute-phase to convalescent-phase samples confirms the diagnosis.[64] Species belonging to the SFG group induce antibodies that cross react with antigens of other group members. The micromethod format of the IFA is an efficient method to test for seroreactive antibodies to several different rickettsial antigens. This method may be useful in areas where several rickettsial species coexist and cause human diseases. The micro-IFA can detect antibodies to up to 9 antigens within a single well containing multiple antigen dots.[65] The serodiagnosis of typhus group rickettsioses is similar to that of RMSF and other SFG rickettsioses.

Another commercially available and fairly sensitive test for RMSF is the ELISA. The subjective nature of reading IFA slides and the requirement for a proficient microscopist is also avoided by using the ELISA technique.[85] Because of the qualitative nature of ELISA, this assay is unable to quantify antibody titers. ELISA is therefore unable to monitor the change in antibody response over time.

Because antibodies against one rickettsial species often cross react with rickettsial antigen from the same group (either SFG or typhus group), conventional methods of serology are unable to serve as a species-specific diagnostic assay. Cross-absorption is performed by separately mixing the serum in question with the different rickettsial antigens involved in the cross reaction. When absorption is performed with the agent responsible for the disease, the homologous and heterologous antibodies are not detected by Western blot. This technique is time consuming and cumbersome when multiple rickettsial agents are in question, but is particularly confounding when the agent is not included in the absorption step or is a novel agent yet to be identified.[88]

In conclusion, seroconversion or a 4-fold increase in titers of IgG from acute-phase to convalescent-phase samples confirms the diagnosis of rickettsial diseases. Detection of rickettsial antigen or nucleic acid by immunohistochemical staining or PCR in biopsy specimens of eschars and papular lesions serves as a reliable assay for early diagnosis. However, clinical manifestations in skin do not occur in every patient. Thus, more reliable, specific, and convenient diagnostic assays are needed for samples such as serum, plasma, and urine.

TREATMENT

Considering the undifferentiated clinical nature of rickettsioses and the usual retrospective fashion in which cases are diagnostically confirmed, knowledge of the epidemiology, signs, and symptoms of rickettsial disease is paramount for the timely empiric administration of effective antimicrobial therapy. Eliciting historical factors such as patient's occupation, travel, recreational activities, and exposure to possible vectors can prompt the inclusion of infection from these agents in the differential diagnosis of an acute febrile illness. This knowledge is key, because antibiotics often used empirically for other infectious syndromes (eg, penicillins, cephalosporins, and sulfonamides) are ineffective against *Rickettsia* spp,[89] and, in the case of sulfonamides, portend poor outcomes.[90]

Tetracyclines are the drug class of choice for the treatment of all SFG and typhus group rickettsioses, with doxycycline being the preferred agent (**Table 3**). The mean inhibitory concentration (MIC) of tetracyclines to *Rickettsia* spp is 0.06 to 0.25 μg/mL.[89] Doxycycline and minocycline have a twice-daily dosing schedule, improved gastrointestinal tolerability, and are bioavailable in the presence of food, which make them superior to tetracycline hydrochloride.[91] Chloramphenicol is generally considered an alternative, with MICs of 0.25 to 2.0 μg/mL,[89,92] but in the most severe rickettsial illness, RMSF, its

Table 3
Treatment of rickettsial diseases

	Medication	Adult Dose	Pediatric Dose	Duration
First choice for virtually all rickettsioses	Doxycycline oral or intravenous[a]	100 mg twice daily	2.2 mg/kg (maximum 100 mg) twice daily	≥3 d after defervescence (minimum course 5–7 d)[b]
Severe RMSF or other severe rickettsial illness[a]	Doxycycline intravenous	200-mg loading dose followed by 100 mg twice daily	2.2 mg/kg (maximum 100 mg) twice daily	≥3 d after defervescence (minimum course 5–7 d)[b]
Alternative for RMSF and other rickettsioses[c]	Chloramphenicol oral or intravenous	500 mg every 6 h	12.5 mg/kg every 6 h	≥3 d after defervescence (minimum course 5–7 d)[b]
Alternative for MSF and other less severe SFG rickettsioses	Oral fluoroquinolones: • Ciprofloxacin • Levofloxacin Oral macrolides: • Clarithromycin • Azithromycin	• 500 mg twice daily • 500 mg daily • 500 mg twice daily • 500 mg daily • 500 mg × 1 then 250 mg daily	• Not recommended • Not recommended • 7.5 mg/kg twice daily • 10 mg/kg daily • 10 mg/kg × 1 then 5 mg/kg daily	 • 5–7 d • 7 d • 3 d • 5 d
Alternative for epidemic louse-borne typhus[d]	Short-course oral doxycycline	200 mg once		
Alternative for murine typhus	Oral fluoroquinolones: • Ciprofloxacin • Levofloxacin	• 500 mg twice daily • 500 mg daily	• Not recommended • Not recommended	5–7 d

[a] The bioavailability of doxycycline is excellent. The decision to choose the parenteral form should be made if gastrointestinal upset precludes its oral use or if absorption is thought to be compromised during critical illness.
[b] The duration of treatment of RMSF is based on experience, because there are no controlled trials to guide the optimal duration.
[c] Chloramphenicol is inferior to doxycycline for RMSF. Its oral form is not available in the United States and the parenteral form is exceedingly hard for hospital pharmacies to stock. It is also associated with gray baby syndrome in neonates and aplastic anemia.
[d] Relapses have been documented. Only recommended if needed for mass treatment to curtail an outbreak, and if medications are in limited supply.

use is associated with a higher case fatality rate than the use of tetracyclines.[93] In a milder illness, murine typhus, chloramphenicol is associated with a longer time to defervesce.[94] Although available in much of the world, oral chloramphenicol is not available in the United States, and the parenteral formulation is becoming increasingly scarce.

There are no clinically evaluated alternatives to doxycycline or chloramphenicol for use in RMSF for which efficacy is supported by vast clinical experience. For MSF, a generally less severe illness than RMSF, clinical studies have been performed to help guide the use of shorter courses of antibiotics[95,96] and alternative agents (see **Table 3**). In less severe illness, fluoroquinolones are effective and have better gastrointestinal tolerance than tetracyclines.[97] However, a report of severe forms of illness associated with their use has tempered their use as a preferred agent.[98] Fluoroquinolones are contraindicated during pregnancy and for routine use in children.

Although the aforementioned antibiotics are orally bioavailable, nausea, vomiting, and critical illness may necessitate hospitalization and use of parenteral formulations. Long or frequent courses of tetracyclines cause staining of permanent teeth in children, but short courses do not appreciably stain teeth,[99,100] and treatment with doxycycline has not been associated with staining of teeth and is therefore recommended for children with a rickettsial illness.[64] Management of pregnant women with RMSF is extremely challenging. Tetracyclines deposit within the fetal skeleton and may cause temporary inhibition of bone growth.[101] They are also associated with maternal hepatotoxicity and pancreatitis.[102] In later pregnancy, transplacental chloramphenicol concentration is theoretically high enough to cause gray baby syndrome (abdominal distention, pallor, cyanosis, and vasomotor collapse).[103] In the United States, weighing the risk/benefit ratios of either drug may be precluded by the limited availability of parenteral chloramphenicol. In pregnant women with less severe illness caused by other rickettsioses, azithromycin may be considered a safe but untested alternative. In those with RMSF and a history of severe hypersensitivity to doxycycline, desensitization is warranted.[104,105]

REFERENCES

1. Yu X-J, Walker DH, Family I. Rickettsiaceae. In: Brenner DJ, Kreig NR, Stanley JT, editors. Bergey's manual of systematic bacteriology, vol. 2, 2nd edition. New York: Springer; 2005. p. 96–116.

2. Ricketts HT. The study of "Rocky Mountain spotted fever" (tick fever?) by means of animal inoculations. JAMA 1906;47:33–6.

3. Ricketts HT. A micro-organism which apparently has a specific relationship to Rocky Mountain spotted fever. JAMA 1909;52:379–80.

4. Wolbach SB, Todd JL, Palfrey FW. The etiology and pathology of typhus. Cambridge (MA): Harvard University Press; 1922.

5. Shankman B. Report on an outbreak of endemic febrile illness, not yet identified, occurring in New York City. N Y State J Med 1946;46:2156–9.

6. Huebner RJ, Stamps P, Armstrong C. Rickettsialpox; a newly recognized rickettsial disease; isolation of the etiological agent. Public Health Rep 1946;61(45):1605–14.

7. Uchida T, Uchiyama T, Kumano K, et al. Rickettsia japonica sp. nov., the etiological agent of spotted fever group rickettsiosis in Japan. Int J Syst Bacteriol 1992;42(2):303–5.

8. Stenos J, Roux V, Walker D, et al. Rickettsia honei sp. nov., the aetiological agent of Flinders Island spotted fever in Australia. Int J Syst Bacteriol 1998;48(Pt 4):1399–404.

9. Paddock CD, Sumner JW, Comer JA, et al. *Rickettsia parkeri*: a newly recognized cause of spotted fever rickettsiosis in the United States. Clin Infect Dis 2004;38(6):805–11.

10. Shapiro MR, Fritz CL, Tait K, et al. Rickettsia 364D: a newly recognized cause of eschar-associated illness in California. Clin Infect Dis 2010;50(4):541–8.

11. Fournier PE, Gouriet F, Brouqui P, et al. Lymphangitis-associated rickettsiosis, a new rickettsiosis caused by *Rickettsia sibirica* mongolotimonae: seven new cases and review of the literature. Clin Infect Dis 2005;40(10):1435–44.

12. Raoult D, Lakos A, Fenollar F, et al. Spotless rickettsiosis caused by *Rickettsia slovaca* and associated with *Dermacentor* ticks. Clin Infect Dis 2002;34(10): 1331–6.

13. Perlman SJ, Hunter MS, Zchori-Fein E. The emerging diversity of *Rickettsia*. Proc Biol Sci 2006;273(1598):2097–106.

14. Niebylski ML, Schrumpf ME, Burgdorfer W, et al. *Rickettsia peacockii* sp. nov., a new species infecting wood ticks, *Dermacentor andersoni*, in western Montana. Int J Syst Bacteriol 1997;47(2):446–52.

15. Kurtti TJ, Felsheim RF, Burkhardt NY, et al. *Rickettsia buchneri* sp. nov., a rickettsial endosymbiont of the blacklegged tick *Ixodes scapularis*. Int J Syst Evol Microbiol 2015;65(Pt 3):965–70.

16. Vitale G, Mansuelo S, Rolain JM, et al. *Rickettsia massiliae* human isolation. Emerg Infect Dis 2006;12(1):174–5.

17. Dahlgren FS, Paddock CD, Springer YP, et al. Expanding range of *Amblyomma americanum* and simultaneous changes in the epidemiology of spotted fever group rickettsiosis in the United States. Am J Trop Med Hyg 2016;94(1):35–42.

18. Walker DH, Paddock CD, Dumler JS. Emerging and re-emerging tick-transmitted rickettsial and ehrlichial infections. Med Clin North Am 2008;92(6): 1345–61, x.

19. Fournier PE, Dumler JS, Greub G, et al. Gene sequence-based criteria for identification of new rickettsia isolates and description of *Rickettsia heilongjiangensis* sp. nov. J Clin Microbiol 2003;41(12):5456–65.

20. Medini D, Serruto D, Parkhill J, et al. Microbiology in the post-genomic era. Nat Rev Microbiol 2008;6(6):419–30.

21. Achtman M, Wagner M. Microbial diversity and the genetic nature of microbial species. Nat Rev Microbiol 2008;6(6):431–40.

22. Gillespie JJ, Williams K, Shukla M, et al. *Rickettsia* phylogenomics: unwinding the intricacies of obligate intracellular life. PLoS One 2008;3(4):e2018.

23. Walker DH, Ismail N. Emerging and re-emerging rickettsioses: endothelial cell infection and early disease events. Nat Rev Microbiol 2008;6(5):375–86.

24. Burgdorfer W. Ecological and epidemiological considerations of Rocky Mountain spotted fever and scrub typhus. In: Walker DH, editor. Biology of rickettsial diseases, vol. 1. Boca Raton (FL): CRC Press; 1988. p. 33–50.

25. Stromdahl EY, Jiang J, Vince M, et al. Infrequency of *Rickettsia rickettsii* in *Dermacentor variabilis* removed from humans, with comments on the role of other human-biting ticks associated with spotted fever group rickettsiae in the United States. Vector Borne Zoonotic Dis 2011;11(7):969–77.

26. Guedes E, Leite RC, Prata MC, et al. Detection of *Rickettsia rickettsii* in the tick *Amblyomma cajennense* in a new Brazilian spotted fever-endemic area in the state of Minas Gerais. Mem Inst Oswaldo Cruz 2005;100(8):841–5.

27. Pinter A, Labruna MB. Isolation of *Rickettsia rickettsii* and *Rickettsia bellii* in cell culture from the tick *Amblyomma aureolatum* in Brazil. Ann N Y Acad Sci 2006; 1078:523–9.

28. Jensenius M, Fournier PE, Kelly P, et al. African tick bite fever. Lancet Infect Dis 2003;3(9):557–64.
29. Fuller HS, Murray ES, Ayres JC, et al. Studies of rickettsialpox. I. Recovery of the causative agent from house mice in Boston, Massachusetts. Am J Hyg 1951; 54(1):82–100.
30. Bechah Y, Capo C, Mege JL, et al. Epidemic typhus. Lancet Infect Dis 2008; 8(7):417–26.
31. Civen R, Ngo V. Murine typhus: an unrecognized suburban vectorborne disease. Clin Infect Dis 2008;46(6):913–8.
32. Sonenshine DE, Bozeman FM, Williams MS, et al. Epizootiology of epidemic typhus (*Rickettsia prowazekii*) in flying squirrels. Am J Trop Med Hyg 1978;27(2 Pt 1):339–49.
33. McDade JE. Flying squirrels and their ectoparasites: disseminators of epidemic typhus. Parasitol Today 1987;3(3):85–7.
34. Medina-Sanchez A, Bouyer DH, Alcantara-Rodriguez V, et al. Detection of a typhus group *Rickettsia* in *Amblyomma* ticks in the state of Nuevo Leon, Mexico. Ann N Y Acad Sci 2005;1063:327–32.
35. Reiss-Gutfreund RJ. The isolation of *Rickettsia prowazeki* and *mooseri* from unusual sources. Am J Trop Med Hyg 1966;15(6):943–9.
36. Demma LJ, Traeger MS, Nicholson WL, et al. Rocky Mountain spotted fever from an unexpected tick vector in Arizona. N Engl J Med 2005;353(6):587–94.
37. Helmick CG, Bernard KW, D'Angelo LJ. Rocky Mountain spotted fever: clinical, laboratory, and epidemiological features of 262 cases. J Infect Dis 1984;150(4): 480–8.
38. Eloubeidi MA, Burton CS, Sexton DJ. The great imitator: Rocky Mountain spotted fever occurring after hospitalization for unrelated illnesses. South Med J 1997;90(9):943–5.
39. Kaplowitz LG, Fischer JJ, Sparling PF. Rocky Mountain spotted fever: a clinical dilemma. In: Remington JB, Swartz HN, editors. Current clinical topics in infectious diseases, vol. 2. New York: McGraw-Hill; 1981. p. 89–108.
40. Kirkland KB, Marcom PK, Sexton DJ, et al. Rocky Mountain spotted fever complicated by gangrene: report of six cases and review. Clin Infect Dis 1993;16(5):629–34.
41. Parola P, Paddock CD, Socolovschi C, et al. Update on tick-borne rickettsioses around the world: a geographic approach. Clin Microbiol Rev 2013;26(4): 657–702.
42. Raoult D, Weiller PJ, Chagnon A, et al. Mediterranean spotted fever: clinical, laboratory and epidemiological features of 199 cases. Am J Trop Med Hyg 1986;35(4):845–50.
43. Paddock CD, Finley RW, Wright CS, et al. *Rickettsia parkeri* rickettsiosis and its clinical distinction from Rocky Mountain spotted fever. Clin Infect Dis 2008; 47(9):1188–96.
44. Parola P, Rovery C, Rolain JM, et al. *Rickettsia slovaca* and *R. raoultii* in tick-borne rickettsioses. Emerg Infect Dis 2009;15(7):1105–8.
45. Umulisa I, Omolo J, Muldoon KA, et al. A mixed outbreak of epidemic typhus fever and trench fever in a youth rehabilitation center: risk factors for illness from a case-control study, Rwanda, 2012. Am J Trop Med Hyg 2016;95(2): 452–6.
46. Raoult D, Ndihokubwayo JB, Tissot-Dupont H, et al. Outbreak of epidemic typhus associated with trench fever in Burundi. Lancet 1998;352(9125):353–8.

47. Perine PL, Chandler BP, Krause DK, et al. A clinico-epidemiological study of epidemic typhus in Africa. Clin Infect Dis 1992;14(5):1149–58.
48. Brill NE. An acute infectious disease of unknown origin; a clinical study based on 221 cases. Am J Med 1952;13(5):533–41.
49. Duma RJ, Sonenshine DE, Bozeman FM, et al. Epidemic typhus in the United States associated with flying squirrels. JAMA 1981;245(22):2318–23.
50. Dumler JS, Taylor JP, Walker DH. Clinical and laboratory features of murine typhus in south Texas, 1980 through 1987. JAMA 1991;266(10):1365–70.
51. Stuart BM, Pullen RL. Endemic (murine) typhus fever: clinical observations of 180 cases. Ann Intern Med 1945;23:17.
52. Blanton LS, Lea AS, Kelly BC, et al. An unusual cutaneous manifestation in a patient with murine typhus. Am J Trop Med Hyg 2015;93:1164–7.
53. Andrew R, Bonnin JM, Williams S. Tick typhus in North Queensland. Med J Aust 1946;2:253–8.
54. Brown LD, Macaluso KR. *Rickettsia felis*, an emerging flea-borne rickettsiosis. Curr Trop Med Rep 2016;3:27–39.
55. Greenberg M, Pellitteri O, Klein IF, et al. Rickettsialpox; a newly recognized rickettsial disease; clinical observations. J Am Med Assoc 1947;133(13):901–6.
56. Kass EM, Szaniawski WK, Levy H, et al. Rickettsialpox in a New York city hospital, 1980 to 1989. N Engl J Med 1994;331(24):1612–7.
57. Walker DH, Feng HM, Ladner S, et al. Immunohistochemical diagnosis of typhus rickettsioses using an anti-lipopolysaccharide monoclonal antibody. Mod Pathol 1997;10:1038–42.
58. Walker DH, Parks FM, Betz TG, et al. Histopathology and immunohistologic demonstration of the distribution of *Rickettsia typhi* in fatal murine typhus. Am J Clin Pathol 1989;91:720–4.
59. Paddock CD, Zaki SR, Koss T, et al. Rickettsialpox in New York City: a persistent urban zoonosis. Ann N Y Acad Sci 2003;990:36–44.
60. Lepidi H, Fournier PE, Raoult D. Histologic features and immunodetection of African tick-bite fever eschar. Emerg Infect Dis 2006;12(9):1332–7.
61. Walker DH. Rocky Mountain spotted fever: a seasonal alert. Clin Infect Dis 1995; 20:1111–7.
62. Rutherford JS, Macaluso KR, Smith N, et al. Fatal spotted fever rickettsiosis, Kenya. Emerg Infect Dis 2004;10(5):910–3.
63. Paddock CD, Greer PW, Ferebee TL, et al. Hidden mortality attributable to Rocky Mountain spotted fever: immunohistochemical detection of fatal, serologically unconfirmed disease. J Infect Dis 1999;179(6):1469–76.
64. Chapman AS, Bakken JS, Folk SM, et al, Tickborne Rickettsial Diseases Working Group, CDC. Diagnosis and management of tickborne rickettsial diseases: Rocky Mountain spotted fever, ehrlichioses, and anaplasmosis—United States: a practical guide for physicians and other health-care and public health professionals. MMWR Recomm Rep 2006;55(RR-4):1–27.
65. La Scola B, Raoult D. Laboratory diagnosis of rickettsioses: current approaches to diagnosis of old and new rickettsial diseases. J Clin Microbiol 1997;35: 2715–27.
66. Denison AM, Amin BD, Nicholson WL, et al. Detection of *Rickettsia rickettsii*, *Rickettsia parkeri*, and *Rickettsia akari* in skin biopsy specimens using a multiplex real-time polymerase chain reaction assay. Clin Infect Dis 2014;59(5): 635–42.

67. Sexton DJ, Kanj SS, Wilson K, et al. The use of a polymerase chain reaction as a diagnostic test for Rocky Mountain spotted fever. Am J Trop Med Hyg 1994;50: 59–63.

68. Mouffok N, Socolovschi C, Benabdellah A, et al. Diagnosis of rickettsioses from eschar swab samples, Algeria. Emerg Infect Dis 2011;17:1968–9.

69. Kondo M, Akachi S, Kawano M, et al. Improvement in early diagnosis of Japanese spotted fever by using a novel Rick PCR system. J Dermatol 2015;42(11): 1066–71.

70. Znazen A, Sellami H, Elleuch E, et al. Comparison of two quantitative real time PCR assays for *Rickettsia* detection in patients from Tunisia. PLoS Negl Trop Dis 2015;9(2):e0003487.

71. Levin ML, Snellgrove AN, Zemtsova GE. Comparative value of blood and skin samples for diagnosis of spotted fever group rickettsial infection in model animals. Ticks Tick Borne Dis 2016;7(5):1029–34.

72. Kato CY, Chung IH, Robinson LK, et al. Assessment of real-time PCR assay for detection of *Rickettsia* spp. and *Rickettsia rickettsii* in banked clinical samples. J Clin Microbiol 2013;51:314–7.

73. Ergas D, Sthoeger ZM, Keysary A, et al. Early diagnosis of severe Mediterranean spotted fever cases by nested-PCR detecting spotted fever Rickettsiae 17-kD common antigen gene. Scand J Infect Dis 2008;40(11–12):965–7.

74. Pan L, Zhang L, Wang G, et al. Rapid, simple, and sensitive detection of the *ompB* gene of spotted fever group rickettsiae by loop-mediated isothermal amplification. BMC Infect Dis 2012;12:254.

75. Tzianabos T, Anderson BE, McDade JE. Detection of *Rickettsia rickettsii* DNA in clinical specimens by using polymerase chain reaction technology. J Clin Microbiol 1989;27:2866–8.

76. Roux V, Raoult D. Phylogenetic analysis of members of the genus *Rickettsia* using the gene encoding the outer-membrane protein rOmpB (*ompB*). Int J Syst Evol Microbiol 2000;50:1449–55.

77. Regnery RL, Spruill CL, Plikaytis BD. Genotypic identification of rickettsiae and estimation of intraspecies sequence divergence for portions of two rickettsial genes. J Bacteriol 1991;173:1576–89.

78. Eremeeva M, Yu X, Raoult D. Differentiation among spotted fever group rickettsiae species by analysis of restriction fragment length polymorphism of PCR-amplified DNA. J Clin Microbiol 1994;32:803–10.

79. Boostrom A, Beier MS, Macaluso JA, et al. Geographic association of *Rickettsia felis*-infected opossums with human murine typhus, Texas. Emerg Infect Dis 2002;8:549–54.

80. Roux V, Fournier PE, Raoult D. Differentiation of spotted fever group rickettsiae by sequencing and analysis of restriction fragment length polymorphism of PCR-amplified DNA of the gene encoding the protein rOmpA. J Clin Microbiol 1996;34:2058–65.

81. Peniche-Lara G, Zavala-Velazquez J, Dzul-Rosado K, et al. Simple method to differentiate among *Rickettsia* species. J Mol Microbiol Biotechnol 2013;23: 203–8.

82. Segura F, Pons I, Sanfeliu I, et al. Shell-vial culture, coupled with real-time PCR, applied to *Rickettsia conorii* and *Rickettsia massiliae*-Bar29 detection, improving the diagnosis of the Mediterranean spotted fever. Ticks Tick Borne Dis 2016;7(3):457–61.

83. Segura F, Pons I, Pla J, et al. Shell-vial culture and real-time PCR applied to *Rickettsia typhi* and *Rickettsia felis* detection. World J Microbiol Biotechnol 2015; 31(11):1747–54.

84. La Scola B, Raoult D. Diagnosis of Mediterranean spotted fever by cultivation of *Rickettsia conorii* from blood and skin samples using the centrifugation-shell vial technique and by detection of *R. conorii* in circulating endothelial cells: a 6-year follow-up. J Clin Microbiol 1996;34(11):2722–7.

85. Clements ML, Dumler JS, Fiset P, et al. Serodiagnosis of Rocky Mountain spotted fever: comparison of IgM and IgG enzyme-linked immunosorbent assays and indirect fluorescent antibody test. J Infect Dis 1983;148:876–80.

86. Jensenius M, Fournier PE, Vene S, et al. Comparison of immunofluorescence, Western blotting, and cross-adsorption assays for diagnosis of African tick bite fever. Clin Diagn Lab Immunol 2004;11(4):786–8.

87. Kaplan JE, Schonberger LB. The sensitivity of various serologic tests in the diagnosis of Rocky Mountain spotted fever. Am J Trop Med Hyg 1986;35:840–4.

88. La Scola B, Rydkina L, Ndihokubwayo JB, et al. Serological differentiation of murine typhus and epidemic typhus using cross-adsorption and Western blotting. Clin Diagn Lab Immunol 2000;7:612–6.

89. Rolain JM, Maurin M, Vestris G, et al. In vitro susceptibilities of 27 rickettsiae to 13 antimicrobials. Antimicrob Agents Chemother 1998;42(7):1537–41.

90. Ruiz Beltran R, Herrero Herrero JI. Deleterious effect of trimethoprim-sulfamethoxazole in Mediterranean spotted fever. Antimicrob Agents Chemother 1992;36(6):1342–3.

91. Moffa M, Brook I. Tetracyclines, glycyclines, and chloramphenicol. In: Bennett JE, Dolin R, Blaser MJ, editors. Mandell, Douglas, and Bennett's principles and practice of infectious diseases, vol. 1, 8th edition. Philadelphia: Elsevier Saunders; 2015. p. 322–38.

92. Raoult D, Drancourt M. Antimicrobial therapy of rickettsial diseases. Antimicrob Agents Chemother 1991;35(12):2457–62.

93. Holman RC, Paddock CD, Curns AT, et al. Analysis of risk factors for fatal Rocky Mountain spotted fever: evidence for superiority of tetracyclines for therapy. J Infect Dis 2001;184(11):1437–44.

94. Gikas A, Doukakis S, Pediaditis J, et al. Comparison of the effectiveness of five different antibiotic regimens on infection with *Rickettsia typhi*: therapeutic data from 87 cases. Am J Trop Med Hyg 2004;70(5):576–9.

95. Bella-Cueto F, Font-Creus B, Segura-Porta F, et al. Comparative, randomized trial of one-day doxycycline versus 10-day tetracycline therapy for Mediterranean spotted fever. J Infect Dis 1987;155(5):1056–8.

96. Yagupsky P, Gross EM, Alkan M, et al. Comparison of two dosage schedules of doxycycline in children with rickettsial spotted fever. J Infect Dis 1987;155(6):1215–9.

97. Ruiz Beltran R, Herrero Herrero JI. Evaluation of ciprofloxacin and doxycycline in the treatment of Mediterranean spotted fever. Eur J Clin Microbiol Infect Dis 1992;11(5):427–31.

98. Botelho-Nevers E, Rovery C, Richet H, et al. Analysis of risk factors for malignant Mediterranean spotted fever indicates that fluoroquinolone treatment has a deleterious effect. J Antimicrob Chemother 2011;66(8):1821–30.

99. Grossman ER, Walchek A, Freedman H. Tetracyclines and permanent teeth: the relation between dose and tooth color. Pediatrics 1971;47(3):567–70.

100. Todd SR, Dahlgren FS, Traeger MS, et al. No visible dental staining in children treated with doxycycline for suspected Rocky Mountain spotted fever. J Pediatr 2015;166(5):1246–51.
101. Cohlan SQ. Teratogenic agents and congenital malformations. J Pediatr 1963; 63:650–9.
102. Herbert WN, Seeds JW, Koontz WL, et al. Rocky Mountain spotted fever in pregnancy: differential diagnosis and treatment. South Med J 1982;75(9):1063–6.
103. Ross S, Burke FG, Sites J, et al. Placental transmission of chloramphenicol (Chloromycetin). J Am Med Assoc 1950;142(17):1361.
104. Fernando SL, Hudson BJ. Rapid desensitization to doxycycline. Ann Allergy Asthma Immunol 2013;111(1):73–4.
105. Stollings JL, Chadha SN, Paul AM, et al. Doxycycline desensitization for a suspected case of ehrlichiosis. J Allergy Clin Immunol Pract 2014;2(1):103–4.

Printed and bound by CPI Group (UK) Ltd, Croydon, CR0 4YY

03/10/2024

01040397-0014